Aqua Aerobics Today

Aqua Aerobics Today!

Carole Casten, Ph.D.
California State University
Dominguez Hills

Series Editor for West's Physical Activities Series

Robert J. O'Connor, Ed.D.
Los Angeles Pierce College

West Publishing Company
Minneapolis/St. Paul   New York   Los Angeles   San Francisco

Cover Photo: Ken Bondy
Text Photos: Ken Bondy
Composition: Patti Zeman
Computer
Illustration/Production: Miyake Illustration & Design

Additional Photos:
David Hanover Photography (pp. 19, 20, 21, 23, 25, 48, 124, 125, 126)
Tom McCarthy/PhotoEdit (p. 51)
David Young-Wolff/PhotoEdit (p. 207)
Tracy Frankel for SHAPE Magazine, August, 1992 (p. 149)

WEST'S COMMITMENT TO THE ENVIRONMENT
In 1906, West Publishing Company began recycling materials left over from the
production of books. This began a tradition of efficient and responsible use of
resources. Today, up to 95 percent of our legal books and 70 percent of our
college and school texts are printed on recycled, acid-free stock. West also
recycles nearly 22 million pounds of scrap paper annually—the equivalent of
181,717 trees. Since the 1960s, West has devised ways to capture and recycle
waste inks, solvents, oils, and vapors created in the printing process. We also
recycle plastics of all kinds, wood, glass, corrugated cardboard, and batteries,
and have eliminated the use of styrofoam book packaging. We at West are
proud of the longevity and the scope of our commitment to the environment.

*PRINTED ON 10% POST
CONSUMER RECYCLED PAPER*

Copyright © 1994   By WEST PUBLISHING COMPANY
                       610 Opperman Drive
                       P.O. Box 64526
                       St. Paul, MN 55164-0526

Printed in the United States of America

01 00 99 98 97 96 95 94   8 7 6 5 4 3 2 1 0

Library of Congress Cataloging-In-Publication Data

Casten, Carole M. Sokolow.
    Aqua aerobics today / Carole Casten.
    p. cm.—(West's physical activities series)
    Includes index.
    ISBN 0-314-93454-5
    1. Aquatic exercises.   2. Aerobics.   I. Title.   II. Series.
GV838.53.E94C37   1994
613.7'1—dc20

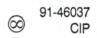

91-46037
CIP

Table of Contents

Preface

AQUA AEROBICS TODAY is designed to supplement your knowledge of aqua aerobics and fitness. The text describes the benefits of aquatic exercise for participants at all levels, from the inexperienced to the advanced. Careful attention has been paid to laying the foundation for a safe, successful, fun, and varied aquatic exercise routine. In addition, the text includes information pertinent to nutrition and weight control, pregnancy and exercise, motivation and the mental aspects of exercising, aqua physics, choreography, and the use of equipment to supplement an aquatic workout. The text also presents information for would-be instructors.

Extensive photographs clearly demonstrate how properly to perform the movements and exercises described in the text. These exercises have been judged physically sound by exercise physiologists and are recognized by highly respected professionals in the field.

The author hopes AQUA AEROBICS TODAY will be a useful tool as you make aquatic exercise a regular part of your life.

To a healthy and fit life!

Acknowledgements

The author is indebted to a number of experts whose contributions to AQUA AEROBICS TODAY have ensured that its content is accurate and on the cutting edge. The author wishes to thank the following: Patricia Mirandy, M.S., for contributing most of the material for the chapter on deep water workouts; Peg Jordan, R.N., co-author of AEROBICS TODAY, for material used in this textbook; Richard Casten, Ph.D., for his contributions, review of the chapter on aqua physics, and unlimited computer technology consulting; Russell Richardson, Ph.D., for his contributions to the exercise physiology content; Ruth Sova, for her innovative thinking and for giving aqua aerobics national attention and recognition; Mary Sanders, for her creative approach to teaching aqua aerobics, her professionalism, her collegiality, and her generosity in sharing photos; Gregory Rosen, M.D., for consulting on pregnancy exercise; Dennis Nowack, D.C., for his contributions to the arthritis content; Julie See, for contributing the choreographed routines (Glenn Miller Medley Routine and Pink Cadillac Routine); and Daniel Berney, M.F.A., for reviewing the aquatic exercise chapter in its early stages. The development of this text could not have progressed without the good advice, shared information, and timely responses of the contributors and reviewers.

The author would like to thank the following colleagues, who offered their expertise and input as complete text reviewers:

Patsy Baird
Texas Wesleyan University

Richard J. Firman, Jr.
California Polytechnic State University

Pauline Foord
Aqua-X Enterprises, California

Freeta Jones
Central State University

Teri MacDonald
Mount Royal College

Marcia Mackey
Temple University

Pat Mirandy
University of Alabama, Huntsville

Jeff Nelken
YMCA of Central Louisiana

Jorge Olaves
Rattler Aquatic Center, Florida

Margot Ross
Mount Royal College

Julie See
Total Workout Center, West Virginia

Dot Shields
University of Florida

Peggy Whilden
Vienna, VA

Ann Wieser
University of North Carolina

Thanks and appreciation is extended to the staff at West Educational Publishing, particularly to Karen Ralling for her hard work and good nature in helping this project become a book and Theresa O'Dell for her confidence in me and her hard work and support in the development and completion of AQUA AEROBICS TODAY.

Sincere gratitude and thanks is extended to the models used throughout this textbook for their good nature, humor, and cooperativeness: Carlos Concetti, Joel Crandall, Kip McClure, Greg Nelson, Karen Shintaku, Karen Vail, Maria Nilsson, Tim Plough, Renee Forrette, Florinda Tamada, Thyme Lewis, Laurie Botwinick, and Tom Smith. Special thanks is also given to the cover models: Bill Addington, Carlos Concetti, Wayne Cropser, Joel Crandall, Toni DiSalvo, James Kamada, Christine Laguna, Kendra Lince, Kip McClure, Mae Isaac McConnell, Zoila Mendieta, Greg Nelson, Irene Regatti, Gwen Robinson, Richard Seitz, Karen Shintaku, Karen Vail, John Whitaker, Ann Windes, and Tracey Windes. Finally, sincere gratitude is extended to Ken Bondy, the book's main photographer, for his patience and good humor.

Several companies contributed equipment and photographs which aided in the presentation of many aqua aerobics movements. The companies that deserve sincere thanks and recognition are Aerobic Workbench, BioEnergetics, Danmar, Hydro-Fit, Hydro-Tone, J&B Foam Fabricators, Inc., and Sprint Rothhammer International, Inc.

The author expresses appreciation to The Spectrum Club in Manhattan Beach, California, for the use of its swimming pool for the cover image and for interior photos of an aqua aerobics class in session. Appreciation is also extended to California State University Dominguez Hills for the use of its swimming pool for the majority of the photographs used in the textbook.

Dedication

This book is dedicated with love and respect to my daughter Kimberly, my husband Rich, and my mother, Frances Sokolow. Without their support and patience, this book would not have been possible. I also dedicate this book to my students, friends, and colleagues, who keep me excited about creating new materials and accepting new challenges. Special thanks is extended to my good friend Michelle Rosen for unlimited use of her warm swimming pool to create movements and test equipment on adults and children.

Carole Casten, Ph.D.

The Series Editor for West's
Physical Activities Series

The Series Editor for West's Physical Activities Series is Dr. Bob O'Connor, Los Angeles Pierce College. Dr. O'Connor received his B.S. and M.S. degrees in physical education from UCLA and his doctorate from U.S.C. His 30-year teaching experience includes instruction in physical education courses of tennis, weight training, volleyball, badminton, swimming and various team sports, as well as classes in teaching methods. He brings to the Series a wide range of college coaching experience in areas of swimming, tennis, water polo, and football. Internationally, Dr. O'Connor has been an advisor to several Olympic programs in weight training and swimming. He was among the first to popularize strength training for all athletic events. Dr. O'Connor has written extensively in the fields of physical education and health and is a dedicated advocate of physical education TODAY.

Books in West's Physical Activities Series

Aerobics Today by Carole Casten and Peg Jordan
Aqua Aerobics Today by Carole Casten
Badminton Today by Tariq Wadood and Karlyne Tan
Jazz Dance Today by Lorraine Person and Kimberly Chandler-Vaccaro
Golf Today by J.C. Snead and John Johnson
Racquetball Today by Lynn Adams and Erwin Goldbloom
Swimming and Aquatics Today by Ron Ballatore and William Miller
Tennis Today by Glenn Bassett and William Otta
Volleyball Today by Marv Dunphy and Rod Wilde
Weight Training Today by Robert O'Connor, Jerry Simmons, and
J. Patrick O'Shea

CHAPTER 1

You're Ready for Aqua Aerobics Today!

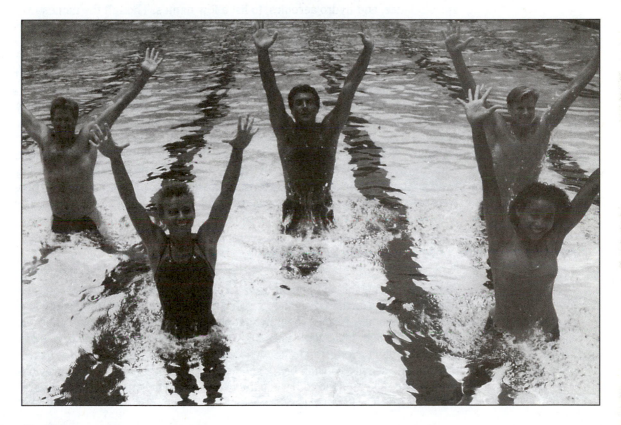

Outline

Overview

If you are looking for a new type of exercise that will leave you feeling exhilarated, then aqua aerobics is your answer! Ease yourself into the pool for a "splashing" time with a stimulating, high-energy workout that, for the most part, is performed in the shallow end of a swimming pool (although some classes include a deep-water workout). Aqua aerobics is also known as aquatic dance exercise, aquatic exercise, water aerobics, water exercise, water workout, splash dance, and hydro aerobics, to list a few names. Though the names may vary, the goal of each class will be similar: to provide you with a fun, high-energy physical conditioning program consisting of continuous, rhythmic movements, usually performed to music in the water, in order to improve your overall fitness level. Aqua aerobics provides an excellent workout for your heart and lungs, and therefore will improve your cardiovascular condition. Aqua aerobics allows you to strengthen and tone your muscles with the effects of gravity greatly reduced. When an exerciser is submerged to neck level, the gravitational pull on the body is reduced by about 90 percent which, in turn, offers an excellent workout environment for almost everyone, including those people who are overweight, pregnant, suffering from a joint problem, or recovering from an injury. Aqua aerobics is a form of exercise that meets the needs of people of all ages and conditions. So ease yourself into the water for aqua aerobics and be on your way to optimal fitness!

Anyone Can Participate in Aqua Aerobics Today!

Anyone can have fun and benefit from taking an aqua aerobics class. Aqua aerobics can be performed by males, females, golden girls, silver men, young people, not-so-young people, healthy people, not-so-healthy people, children, pregnant women, teenagers—actually, *anyone can participate in aqua aerobics today!* You don't even need to know how to swim to benefit from it—aqua aerobics is one activity you can begin and experience success in without previous experience. All you need to have is the desire to participate in a fun, exhilarating exercise class in the water.

People of all ages can participate in aquatic exercise.

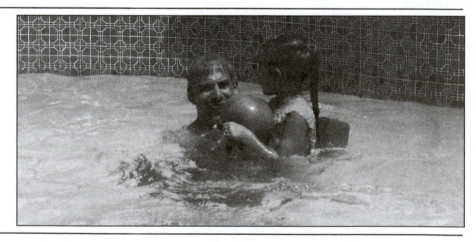

Since the buoyancy of the water supports approximately 70 to 80 percent of your body weight when you are submerged to a level between your nipples and your armpits, you will effectively weigh only 20 to 30 percent of what you do on land. Salt- and mineral-water pools provide even greater density than fresh-water swimming areas, and therefore yield greater buoyancy for your body. So no matter what your present condition, shape, weight, or age, you will be able to perform movements in the water that you never dreamed you could on land. A comprehensive aquatic exercise program, such as the one described in this textbook, includes activities that will work your entire body. These activities will help to firm, tone, and strengthen your muscles, and improve your flexibility as well as your cardiovascular system (heart, lungs, circulation).

Generally, aqua aerobics is performed in the shallow water of a swimming pool; in classes with a deep-water component, buoyancy equipment is used. Hence, even if you do not feel comfortable in the water, you can still enjoy aqua aerobics. Exercisers who are fearful in a water environment may take a position close to the edge of the pool, where they can hold onto the side if they ever lose their step or confidence. Whether in shallow or deep water in your aquatic exercise program, all movements are designed so you never have to submerge your head fully or get your hair wet. If your hair is a concern of yours and you want to make sure that the ends don't get wet from a stray splash, you may want to wear a swimming cap (or a shower cap) during class. This will also save you time after class when getting ready to face the world again.

If you have a medical problem or are concerned about exercising, you should see your physician before beginning the class. Additionally, if you have been sedentary you should have a complete physical examination by your physician before you begin *any* exercise program. Do not fear, however, since almost everyone can benefit from an aqua aerobics class. Since the water provides a cushion for your body during the activities, you should be able to do things you can't do on land, while greatly reducing the risk of injury.

If you are recovering from an injury and concerned about resuming your exercise regime, aquatic exercise is an excellent way to rehabilitate yourself gradually. You will, of course, first want to check with your physician, but chances are that you will be given a prescription of progressive exercise. Aquatic exercise is an excellent way to regain your fitness level and gradually bring mobility, strength, endurance, and flexibility back to injured body parts.

Pool Safety Rules

Swimmers and nonswimmers alike participating in an aqua aerobics class need to pay careful attention to pool safety rules. When you first enter a swimming pool area, look around and distinguish the deep end of the pool from the shallow end. Nonswimmers should enter and remain in the shallow end. All participants should enter the pool by using the steps or ladders or by jumping into the pool feetfirst. *Never* dive headfirst into shallow water—doing so could result in head and neck injuries, or even paralysis. Only dive into a pool with a water depth of eight or more feet.

Before entering the pool, read the pool safety rules and guidelines. Familiarize yourself with the pool safety and rescue equipment. Check the pool area for emergency exits and an emergency phone.

Respect the other people in your class. Never splash others on purpose; no one likes to get wet unnecessarily. Never push others into the swimming pool; doing so could cause an accident. The person you push could hit the pool edge with his/her head or back and sustain a variety of injuries. If the person lands headfirst in the shallow end of the pool, he/she could suffer a serious head or neck injury, possibly even paralysis. Also, do not push someone else under the water. The person may not take a breath before you push and hold him/her under the water, and he/she could pass out due to lack of oxygen. If held under water too long, a person's lungs could fill up with water, and he/she could drown.

It is important for your safety that you wait for the instructor or a certified lifeguard to be on duty in the pool area before you enter the water. Even if you are a good swimmer, you should never swim alone or in an unsupervised area. Accidents do occur and you might need help in case of an emergency. Always walk cautiously on the pool deck. Pool decks are usually wet and often slippery; if you are not careful, you could slip and fall. This could result in a variety of injuries, ranging from mild to serious. It could even result in death—a non-swimmer could slip and fall into the deep end of the pool, becoming a drowning victim.

Never drink alcohol or take recreational drugs prior to class. When inebriated or "high" you do not have complete control over your body, and this could result in an accident or severe injury. When taking prescription drugs, check with your physician before you go to an aqua aerobics class on the medication to make sure it won't impair your coordination and place you in a dangerous situation. It is also advisable to alert the instructor when you are taking medications that could impair your coordination.

Personal Equipment and Supplies

To have fun and obtain the benefits of aqua aerobics you don't need to go out and build yourself a $30,000 swimming pool—all you need to do is find a bathing suit, a pool that offers a class (so you can first learn the activities), a towel, a pair of aquatic exercise shoes, and a good attitude. Aquatic exercise shoes are now produced by several manufacturers and are available in sporting goods stores, discount stores, and department stores at reasonable prices. Aquatic exercise shoes are important to use in an aquatic exercise class because they are made to support your foot and to increase traction on the deck and bottom of the pool.

There are definite advantages to having good-quality aquatic exercise shoes. First of all, these shoes have been designed specifically for the type of class and activities you will be participating in. Second, the soles of these shoes have the proper pattern for providing traction with the pool bottom and will allow you to move safely and efficiently through the water during class. Also, unprotected feet may become irritated from the pool bottom after several days of activities. The traction provided with the pool deck when walking will help to prevent you from slipping and falling before and after class. It will be worth your while to invest in a good pair of aquatic exercise shoes to allow you to obtain the maximum benefits while engaging safely in aqua aerobics.

Good-quality aquatic exercise shoes support the foot and increase traction with the pool deck and bottom.

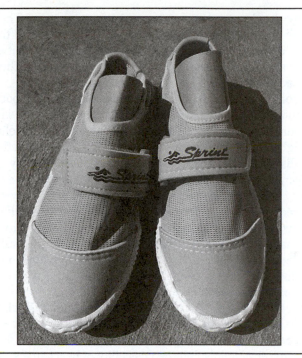

Health Benefits of Aqua Aerobics

Aquatic exercise is well suited to meet the health needs of almost everyone. Working out in the water can be strenuous enough to challenge a highly conditioned athlete as well as a novice. The benefits of aquatic exercise are perfect for all people who want to accomplish an overall body workout in one location without feeling sweat or a jarring impact on their joints. Some people use aqua aerobics as a supplement to other workouts, some use it as a cross-training activity, and still others use aquatic exercise as their only form of exercise.

When exercising, the body eliminates excess heat through perspiration. Even though you may not feel your body sweating during your aquatic workout, you will be working hard, dissipating body heat through perspiration, and achieving the same benefits as from any other form of aerobic exercise such as jogging, aerobic dance, and bicycling. It is important for you to replenish the water in your body *before* you feel thirsty. Hydrating your body while working out will help you maintain maximum energy during your aqua aerobics class and will accelerate your recovery following the class. You need to be sure to drink at least one 8-ounce glass of water before, during, and following an aqua aerobics class. Place a plastic water bottle on the pool edge so that you can sip water during the class whenever you need it.

According to the definition of aerobic exercise, to exercise aerobically your body must use oxygen during a sustained activity of two minutes or longer. An aqua aerobics class will meet that requirement, usually in the first two minutes during a thermal warm-up activity. According to guidelines of the American College of Sports Medicine, in order to gain the greatest aerobic benefit from exercising you should exercise aerobically for 20 to 60 minutes three to five times per week.

Why should you care about exercising aerobically? The benefits of aerobic exercise are numerous. Research has firmly established that regular exercise is beneficial to the human body. One major benefit is that after exercising aerobically an individual feels "good" and exhilarated. Another benefit of aerobic exercise is a reduction of stress and tension in the body.

Aerobic exercise may also reduce some people's blood cholesterol levels. High cholesterol levels have been found to be associated with an increased risk of coronary heart disease. The high proportion of blood cholesterol associated with high-density lipoproteins (HDL) seems to be protective against coronary heart disease, while the opposite is true of low-density lipoproteins (LDL). Coronary risk is lowered by increasing the beneficial type of cholesterol, HDL. The way this works is that about 75 percent of your body's cholesterol is manufactured by the liver. The liver changes the cholesterol into LDLs and triglycerides, which enter the bloodstream and are deposited into various tissues. The LDLs that weren't deposited because the cells were too full leave their cholesterol along arterial walls. The resulting formation of plaque along the arterial walls blocks the bloodstream. Any HDLs in the area will remove excess cholesterol from the bloodstream.

Research has demonstrated that the levels of HDL cholesterol have been found to be higher in people who regularly participate in aerobic exercise. Also, it has been shown that the blood of active individuals has a decreased tendency to clot, thereby diminishing the possibility of heart attack. Recent research has indicated that the relationship between cholesterol and exercise is extremely complex.* For the aforementioned reasons, some authorities are convinced that aerobic-type exercising can help to avert coronary heart disease and help to rehabilitate heart attack victims.

Other benefits of aerobic exercising are that muscle fibers become larger and perform more efficiently. Bones strengthen, become more dense, and are more resistant to deterioration. Aerobic exercising facilitates weight control by raising the metabolic rate, burning additional calories, increasing fat utilization, and improving digestion and elimination. Additionally, the body becomes more physically fit: the heart muscle becomes stronger and more efficient as it pumps more blood with each stroke, lung capacity increases, muscles increase in strength and endurance, and the body becomes more flexible. People who exercise regularly report that they feel better psychologically. Hence, aerobic exercise offers both psychological and physiological benefits.

The benefits of conditioning and overall physical fitness will be discussed in further depth in Chapter 2.

Pool Temperature

Most public swimming pools are kept in the range of 78° to 84° F. A pool at 78° is too cool for an aqua aerobics class. The ideal range for aquatic exercising is 80° to 83°, according to Ruth Sova, president of the Aquatic Exercise Association.** When you first walk into the pool you will feel cool because of

*Kusinitz and Fire, *Your Guide to Getting Fit*, Second Edition.
**Good Health Magazine*, April 28, 1991.

the difference between your natural body temperature and that of the water. But after you've been exercising in the water for about five minutes your core (internal) body temperature will increase, you will adjust to the temperature of the pool, and you will be able to exercise comfortably. If you find that you are getting all the way through the class and are still feeling cold, there are several things you should do. First of all, tell your instructor. Second, ask yourself if you are working to the best of your ability and "giving it your all" (exerting sufficient energy for each movement) during the class. If not, you may need to put more energy into future classes. Finally, a simple solution might be to insulate your body by wearing a T-shirt or other acceptable athletic wear over or under your bathing suit and tights/leggings on your legs. Some people with little tolerance to water temperature wear lightweight, wet suit-type vests over their chests or long-sleeved unitards in the water to aid body insulation.

Practicing Aqua Aerobics

Where and How Can I Practice?

Once you have learned how to participate in aqua aerobics by taking a class, you may ask the question "Where can I practice this activity on my own?" You can do so at any pool that is deep enough for you to stand with your shoulders in the water. This means you can practice in a public pool, in a hotel pool, in your own pool (if you have one)—really, in any swimming pool! Just plan your aqua aerobics workout, have it well in mind, start your music, walk into the pool, and begin.

What Should I Bring with Me?

You don't need very much equipment to prepare yourself to participate in aqua aerobics. Actually, your bag will probably be filled with more toiletries than gear! The personal equipment you will need in order to perform successfully in an aqua aerobics class consists of:

- A bathing suit/bathing trunks.
- A towel.
- Aquatic exercise shoes.
- A swimming cap or a shower cap, if desired, depending on your hair and how much time you have available after class.
- A waterproof sunscreen and/or a hat, and plastic sunglasses, if desired when exercising in an outdoor pool.
- Toiletries.

To work out on your own, you will also need a buddy to act as your lifeguard if there is not one on duty, plus some of the following equipment, depending on your specific workout:

- A cassette tape and a battery-operated cassette tape player.
- Hand paddles or webbed gloves.
- A kickboard.

- Dumbbell-type floats (two empty one-gallon plastic bottles serve in a pinch, but remember that they were *not* designed to be used as aqua aerobics equipment and thus will neither be as safe nor serve you as well as proper equipment).
- Any additional aquatic exercise equipment that you wish to use.

Components of a Class

Since the intention of an aqua aerobics class is to condition your body, the format of each class, regardless of the instructor, will be similar. A class will usually last one hour; however, the class time may vary slightly depending on the facility. All classes you take will have the following general organization:

1. Warm-up/thermal warm-up (5 to 10 minutes).
2. Aqua aerobic activities (15 to 30 minutes).
3. Muscular strength, flexibility, and endurance activities (10 to 20 minutes).
4. Cool-down and stretching (5 minutes).

Every instructor will start the class a little differently. Some instructors like students to walk around the pool area and progressively increase the pace, to give the body a general warm-up. Once the body is warmed up, then land stretches may be performed. Following those activities, the students ease themselves into the pool and begin a class following the formula listed above. Other instructors begin the class in the water and execute all of the warm-ups and stretches there. Both styles are correct; just be aware that there are two philosophies prevailing in teaching aquatic exercise classes.

Patience is Necessary When Learning Aqua Aerobics

No matter what physical activity you are engaging in, it is important that you demonstrate patience during the learning process. You must increase your activity level in a systematic, progressive manner in order to avoid straining yourself in any way or burning out before you've achieved the benefits of exercising. As with any new thing that you are learning, the first day or week may be the most difficult for you. You will need to learn new ways of moving through the water. If you haven't exercised regularly, you may feel a little fatigued following the class. Give yourself a chance—don't be an exercise dropout!

An aqua aerobics class generally consists of a warm-up followed by aqua aerobic activities; muscular strength, flexibility, and endurance activities; and a cool-down.

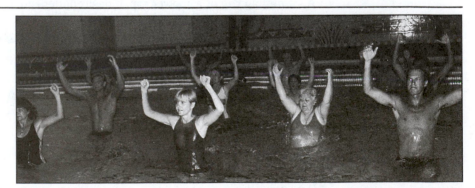

Be patient with yourself when first participating in an aqua aerobics class. During each class, "read" your body signals. If you feel that you are exerting yourself too much, take it easy. Maybe you need to make your movements smaller than those the instructor is demonstrating. Maybe it means you need to go slower. Don't worry if you are "splashing to your own drummer!" The class is for *you* to improve *your* fitness level. This is not a competitive sport; work at your own pace and progress as you see fit for your own body. It is likely that you will feel fatigued at the completion of the class. If you still feel fatigued two hours later, however, it is very possible that you overexerted yourself during class. If you are having the opposite problem—you don't feel that you are exerting yourself enough—perhaps you need to put more energy and power into each movement and increase the size, force, or speed of your movements. Talk to your instructor about this problem before or after class to see if you are understanding all the movements and performing them properly.

Research has shown that aqua aerobics will give you a good workout. A study conducted in 1987 by Whitley and Schoene compared subjects exercising on land (walking on a treadmill) with subjects walking at the same rate in water. The results indicated that the heart rate of the subjects increased 135 percent from their resting level during aquatic walking, compared to only 19 percent when exercising at the same rate on land. Whitley and Schoene also found that the subjects exercising in water increased their heart rate to 75 percent of their maximal heart rate, an intensity sufficient for cardiorespiratory benefits.*

A study conducted by Wigglesworth, Edwards, Mikesky, and Evenbeck demonstrated that water exercise could provide a sufficient workload to elicit cardiorespiratory improvements. A more recent study conducted by Spitzer, Moore, and Hopkins provided evidence that aquatic exercise and low-impact aerobics produced similar training benefits. The aquatic exercisers demonstrated greater strength gains as compared to the low-impact aerobics participants (see Spitzer, Moore, et al in Appendix B).

Summary

1. Aqua aerobics activities are usually performed in shallow water, although some classes include a deep-water component.
2. Aqua aerobics is an activity in which people of all ages and most conditions can participate.
3. When participating in aqua aerobics activities the buoyancy of the water supports 70 to 80 percent of your body weight, so you will effectively weigh only 20 to 30 percent of what you do on land if you are submerged to between the nipple and armpit areas.
4. If you have been sedentary, see your physician for a complete physical examination before beginning any exercise program.
5. If you are recovering from an injury, remember that aqua aerobics may be the perfect activity for you. Water exercise is an excellent way to rehabilitate yourself. Aqua aerobics will help you gradually to bring mobility and strength to injured body parts and help you to regain your previous fitness level.

*J.D. Whitley and L.L. Schoene, "Comparison of Heart Rate Responses: Water Walking versus Treadmill Walking," *Physical Therapy* 67, (1987), pp. 1501–1504.

Checklist: Equipment Needed to Work Out

Before you head off to work out in an aqua aerobics class or in your local pool, be sure you check your equipment against the list below so that when you get there you won't discover that you forgot something and be disappointed.

- Bathing suit/bathing trunks.
- Towel(s).
- Aquatic exercise shoes.
- Webbed gloves or paddles.
- Shampoo.
- Hair dryer.
- Toiletries.
- Music cassette tape.
- Battery-operated cassette player.
- Supplemental aquatic exercise equipment.
- Sunscreen cream and/or a hat if you are working out in an outdoor pool, and plastic sunglasses.

6. Students should follow pool and class safety rules.
7. Aquatic exercise shoes provide support to your feet and traction with the pool bottom and pool deck.
8. Remember that aquatic exercise is a perfect aerobic type of workout. Even though you won't feel your body perspiring while working out in the water, you will be working hard and achieving the same benefits of any other form of aerobic exercise such as jogging, aerobic dance, bicycling, etc.
9. The American College of Sports Medicine guidelines recommend participation in aerobic activities three to five times per week in 20- to 60-minute periods for maximum aerobic benefits.
10. The four components of a class are:

    - Warm-up/thermal warm-up.
    - Aerobic activities.
    - Strength, muscular, and endurance activities.
    - Cool-down, including flexibility movements.

11. Demonstrate patience when learning aqua aerobics.
12. Aquatic exercise and low-impact aerobics produce similar training benefits.

CHAPTER 2

Fitness and Conditioning

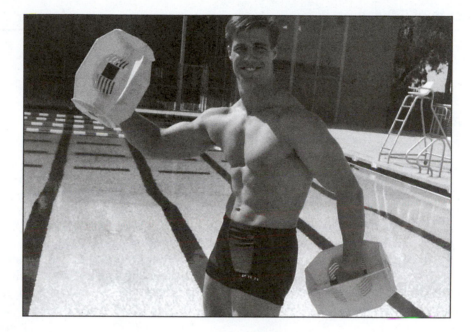

Outline

The benefits of aqua aerobic exercise are numerous, and were described in part in Chapter 1. Research has firmly established that regular exercise is beneficial to the human body. Regular participation in aqua aerobics will help to improve your overall physical fitness level and will probably leave you feeling exhilarated. This chapter will teach you the components of fitness and the principles of conditioning applicable to the benefits you will derive from regular participation in aqua aerobics.

Components of Fitness

There are five components of fitness:

1. Cardiorespiratory endurance and cardiovascular efficiency.
2. Muscular strength.
3. Muscular endurance.
4. Flexibility.
5. Body composition.

An individual is considered to be physically fit when these five components of fitness are developed and balanced. It is important for you to understand these components so that you know what is necessary to keep your body in optimal physical condition.

Your health and quality of life are related to your fitness level. According to recommendations made by the President's Council on Physical Fitness and Sports, a person who is even minimally physically fit has enough strength and endurance to perform daily tasks without undue fatigue, has enough energy left over to enjoy leisure activities, and still is able to deal with an emergency situation.

Component 1: Cardiorespiratory Endurance and Cardiovascular Efficiency

Cardiorespiratory endurance and cardiovascular efficiency, or aerobic fitness, is the ability of the circulatory, respiratory, and vascular systems to deliver blood (and therefore oxygen and nutrients) to the working muscles, cells, and vital organs during prolonged exercise and while at rest. The blood also transports and removes waste products from the muscles, tissues, and vital organs. The cardiorespiratory system consists of the heart and lungs; the vascular system consists of the blood-transporting systems of the body: the arteries, veins, capillaries, and blood vessels. The term *cardiovascular* refers to the heart and the blood-transporting systems of the body.

At all times, but particularly during the stress of exercise, the cardiorespiratory and cardiovascular systems must be able to transport oxygen efficiently to the heart, lungs, working muscles, and tissues in the body, in order to provide the energy required for the body to function. Efficient cardiorespiratory and cardiovascular systems are essential to a high level of physical fitness. Exercise increases the strength of the heart which, in turn, improves the heart's ability to pump blood more efficiently throughout the body.

Cardiovascular and cardiorespiratory endurance are improved and achieved through participation in aerobic activities. Aerobic means "with air," or utilizing oxygen. Aerobic exercise requires large amounts of oxygen transfer during activity over an extended period of time. When an activity is done on a regular basis for an extended period of time, it will improve the heart's pumping ability as well as the circulatory system's ability to transport oxygen more efficiently. Oxygen is inhaled into the lungs, where it is diffused into the blood and carried mostly by the red blood cells to the working muscles and other body parts. Consistent participation in aerobic exercise will improve the body's ability to process oxygen efficiently, which will result in an improvement in aerobic capacity and cardiovascular respiratory endurance. Aerobic activities include (but are not limited to) aqua aerobics, swimming, dance exercise aerobics, bench step aerobics, jogging, cycling, stair climbing, walking, rope jumping, rowing machine activities, and treadmill walking or running.

Anaerobic means "without air." Anaerobic activities are those that involve spurts of power in a starting-and-stopping manner. This includes activities such as tennis, racquetball, and short sprinting activities. In anaerobic activities you are essentially using up oxygen in the body and replacing it later; this action places the body in temporary oxygen debt. Anaerobic activity does not depend on the air you are breathing during exercise, since the duration of the activity is usually less than one minute. For this reason, anaerobic exercise does not improve cardiovascular/cardiorespiratory endurance.

Component 2: Muscular Strength

Muscular strength is the amount of force produced when a muscle group contracts and moves a resistance. A resistance is any amount of additional weight the body moves, including the water. Muscular strength is increased when the muscle is overloaded by repetitive activities and/or when a resistance or weight is added to the muscle action. When you perform exercise overload in a progressive and moderate amount, you strengthen muscles. However, if exercise overload is done in a nonprogressive, uncontrolled, and excessive manner, injury might occur. Strength is essential to a variety of everyday activities such as lifting and moving objects; opening doors, jars, and windows; and carrying children, grocery bags, and luggage. Since water provides 12 times more resistance than air, exercising in the water will help improve your muscular strength.

Component 3: Muscular Endurance

Muscular endurance is the ability of the muscles to exert force over an extended period of time. Endurance is an important element in helping you participate in repetitive activities, such as aqua aerobics, dance exercise, jogging, swimming, walking, and stair climbing.

Component 4: Flexibility

Flexibility is the possible range of motion in each joint, and is necessary to maintain body mobility. The more flexible you are, the more easily you can move your limbs through their full range of motion. The more flexible your muscles are, the fewer sore muscles and joint injuries you will experience. Inactivity can produce the effect of tightening or shortening the muscles, thereby yielding a greater risk of injury when the muscles are put to use or stressed even a little.

Component 5: Body Composition

Body composition is the percentage of total body weight composed of lean body mass (muscle and bones) in relation to the body weight composed of fat tissue. Body composition cannot be measured on a weight scale, but only through hydrostatic weighing (underwater weighing), electrical impedance (measuring a current through the body), skinfold calipers (pinching subcutaneous layers), or circumferential measuring (of waist, thighs, and so on). The American College of Sports Medicine guidelines recommend that you maintain the following percentages of body fat to be considered healthy: men, 15 to 18 percent; women, 20 to 25 percent. To be considered lean, the recommended amounts of body fat for men are 12 to 15 percent; for women, 18 to 22 percent. The recommended percentages change slightly with age. An individual should consult a physician if his/her status is in question.

The amount of fat on the body is determined by the number and size of the fat cells. The size of the cells can be stretched through overeating during any phase of a lifetime. One pound of fat stores about 3,500 calories in a form of liquid fat known as triglyceride. Another important fat in the body is cholesterol, which plays a vital role in heart disease and was discussed in Chapter 1.

Lifestyles and the Development of Cardiovascular Disease

Studies show that certain attributes, habits, and styles of living have a high degree of correlation with the development of cardiovascular disease. Factors known to increase the risks of cardiovascular disease include a family history of heart disease, high blood pressure, cigarette smoking, being overweight, high levels of triglycerides and cholesterol in the blood, diabetes, stress, and physical inactivity.

An analysis of your personal risk factors will guide you toward achieving a healthy lifestyle. To perform a self-analysis, complete the following RISKO Factor Profile.

RISKO Factor Profile

Instructions: To determine your score, circle the appropriate numbers to the right of each item that applies to you. Then add up your score and check your risk analysis against the scoring list.

MEN: Find the column for your age group. Everyone starts with a score of 10 points. Work down the page adding points to your score or subtracting points from your score.

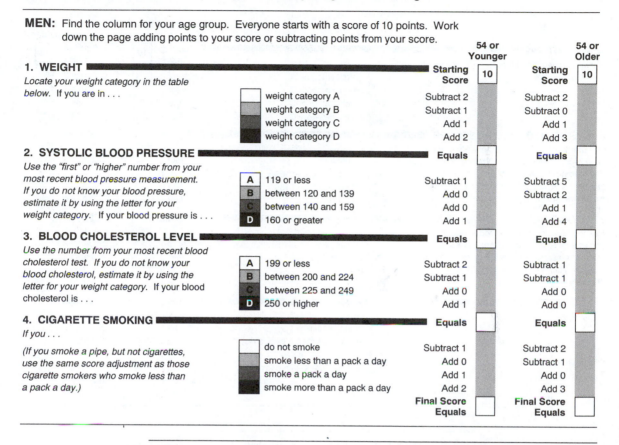

		54 or Younger	54 or Older
1. WEIGHT		**Starting Score** 10	**Starting Score** 10
Locate your weight category in the table below. If you are in . . .	weight category A	Subtract 2	Subtract 2
	weight category B	Subtract 1	Subtract 0
	weight category C	Add 1	Add 1
	weight category D	Add 2	Add 3
2. SYSTOLIC BLOOD PRESSURE		**Equals**	**Equals**
Use the "first" or "higher" number from your most recent blood pressure measurement. If you do not know your blood pressure, estimate it by using the letter for your weight category. If your blood pressure is . . .	A 119 or less	Subtract 1	Subtract 5
	B between 120 and 139	Add 0	Subtract 2
	C between 140 and 159	Add 0	Add 1
	D 160 or greater	Add 1	Add 4
3. BLOOD CHOLESTEROL LEVEL		**Equals**	**Equals**
Use the number from your most recent blood cholesterol test. If you do not know your blood cholesterol, estimate it by using the letter for your weight category. If your blood cholesterol is . . .	A 199 or less	Subtract 2	Subtract 1
	B between 200 and 224	Subtract 1	Subtract 1
	C between 225 and 249	Add 0	Add 0
	D 250 or higher	Add 1	Add 0
4. CIGARETTE SMOKING		**Equals**	**Equals**
If you . . . (If you smoke a pipe, but not cigarettes, use the same score adjustment as those cigarette smokers who smoke less than a pack a day.)	do not smoke	Subtract 1	Subtract 2
	smoke less than a pack a day	Add 0	Subtract 1
	smoke a pack a day	Add 1	Add 0
	smoke more than a pack a day	Add 2	Add 3
		Final Score Equals	**Final Score Equals**

WEIGHT TABLE FOR MEN

Look for your height (without shoes) in the far left column and then read across to find the category into which your weight (in indoor clothing) would fall.

Because both blood pressure and blood cholesterol are related to weight, an estimate of these risk factors for each weight category is printed at the bottom of the table.

Your Height		Weight Category (lbs.)			
Ft.	In.	A	B	C	D
5	1	up to 123	124–148	149–173	174 plus
5	2	up to 126	127–152	153–178	179 plus
5	3	up to 129	130–156	157–182	183 plus
5	4	up to 132	133–160	161–186	187 plus
5	5	up to 135	136–163	164–190	191 plus
5	6	up to 139	140–168	169–196	197 plus
5	7	up to 144	145–174	175–203	204 plus
5	8	up to 148	149–179	180–209	210 plus
5	9	up to 152	153–184	185–214	215 plus
5	10	up to 157	158–190	191–221	222 plus
5	11	up to 161	162–194	195–227	228 plus
6	0	up to 165	166–199	200–232	233 plus
6	1	up to 170	171–205	206–239	240 plus
6	2	up to 175	176–211	212–246	247 plus
6	3	up to 180	181–217	218–253	254 plus
6	4	up to 185	186–223	224–260	261 plus
6	5	up to 190	191–229	230–267	268 plus
6	6	up to 195	196–235	236–274	275 plus
Estimate of Systolic Blood Pressure		119 or less	120 to 139	140 to 159	160 or more
Estimate of Blood Cholesterol		199 or less	200 to 224	225 to 249	250 or more

WOMEN: Find the column for your age group. Everyone starts with a score of 10 points. Work down the page adding points to your score or subtracting points from your score.

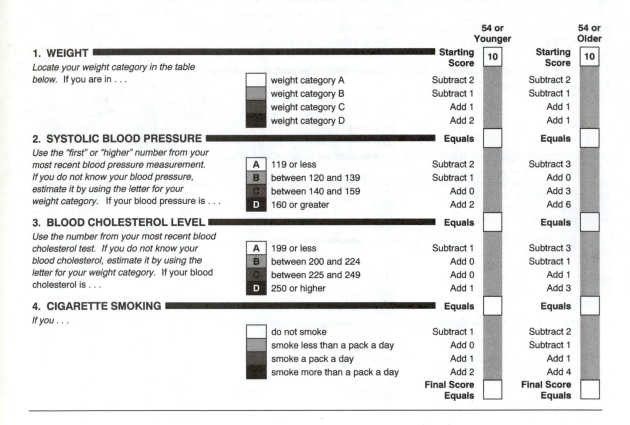

		54 or Younger	54 or Older
1. WEIGHT		**Starting Score** 10	**Starting Score** 10
Locate your weight category in the table below. If you are in . . .			
	weight category A	Subtract 2	Subtract 2
	weight category B	Subtract 1	Subtract 1
	weight category C	Add 1	Add 1
	weight category D	Add 2	Add 1
2. SYSTOLIC BLOOD PRESSURE		**Equals**	**Equals**
Use the "first" or "higher" number from your most recent blood pressure measurement. If you do not know your blood pressure, estimate it by using the letter for your weight category. If your blood pressure is . . .	A 119 or less	Subtract 2	Subtract 3
	B between 120 and 139	Subtract 1	Add 0
	C between 140 and 159	Add 0	Add 3
	D 160 or greater	Add 2	Add 6
3. BLOOD CHOLESTEROL LEVEL		**Equals**	**Equals**
Use the number from your most recent blood cholesterol test. If you do not know your blood cholesterol, estimate it by using the letter for your weight category. If your blood cholesterol is . . .	A 199 or less	Subtract 1	Subtract 3
	B between 200 and 224	Add 0	Subtract 1
	C between 225 and 249	Add 0	Add 1
	D 250 or higher	Add 1	Add 3
4. CIGARETTE SMOKING		**Equals**	**Equals**
If you . . .			
	do not smoke	Subtract 1	Subtract 2
	smoke less than a pack a day	Add 0	Subtract 1
	smoke a pack a day	Add 1	Add 1
	smoke more than a pack a day	Add 2	Add 4
		Final Score Equals	**Final Score Equals**

WEIGHT TABLE FOR WOMEN	Your Height		Weight Category (lbs.)			
	Ft.	In.	A	B	C	D
Look for your height (without shoes) in the far left column and then read across to find the category into which your weight (in indoor clothing) would fall.	4	8	up to 101	102–122	123–143	144 plus
	4	9	up to 103	104–125	126–146	147 plus
	4	10	up to 106	107–128	129–150	151 plus
	4	11	up to 109	110–132	133–154	155 plus
	5	0	up to 112	113–136	137–158	159 plus
	5	1	up to 115	116–139	140–162	163 plus
	5	2	up to 119	120–144	145–168	169 plus
	5	3	up to 122	123–148	149–172	173 plus
	5	4	up to 127	128–154	155–179	180 plus
	5	5	up to 131	132–158	159–185	186 plus
	5	6	up to 135	136–163	164–190	191 plus
	5	7	up to 139	140–168	169–196	197 plus
	5	8	up to 143	144–173	174–202	203 plus
Because both blood pressure and blood cholesterol are related to weight, an estimate of these risk factors for each weight category is printed at the bottom of the table.	5	9	up to 147	148–178	179–207	208 plus
	5	10	up to 151	152–182	183–213	214 plus
	5	11	up to 155	156–187	188–218	219 plus
	6	0	up to 159	160–191	192–224	225 plus
	6	1	up to 163	164–196	197–229	230 plus
Estimate of Systolic Blood Pressure			119 or less	120 to 139	140 to 159	160 or more
Estimate of Blood Cholesterol			199 or less	200 to 224	225 to 249	250 or more

WHAT YOUR SCORE MEANS

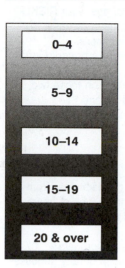

0–4
5–9
10–14
15–19
20 & over

You have one of the lowest risks of heart disease for your age and sex.

You have a low to moderate risk of heart disease for your age and sex, but there is some room for improvement.

You have a moderate to high risk of heart disease for your age and sex, with considerable room for improvement on some factors.

You have a high risk of developing heart disease for your age and sex, with a great deal of room for improvement on all factors.

You have a very high risk of developing heart disease for your age and sex and should take immediate action on all risk factors.

WARNING

- If you do not know your current blood pressure or blood cholesterol level, you should visit your physician or health center to have them measured. Then figure your score again for a more accurate determination of your risk.
- If you are overweight, have high blood pressure or high blood cholesterol, or smoke cigarettes, your long-term risk of heart disease is increased even if your risk in the next several years is low.

HOW TO REDUCE YOUR RISK

- Try to quit smoking permanently. There are many programs available.
- Have your blood pressure checked regularly, preferably every twelve months after age 40. If your blood pressure is high, see your physician. Remember blood pressure medicine is only effective if taken regularly.
- Consider your daily exercise (or lack of it). A half hour of brisk walking, swimming, or other enjoyable activity should not be difficult to fit into your day.
- Give some serious thought to your diet. If you are overweight, or eat a lot of foods high in saturated fat or cholesterol (whole milk, cheese, eggs, butter, fatty foods, fried foods) then changes should be made in your diet. Look for the American Heart Association Cookbook at your local bookstore.
- Visit or write your local Heart Association for further information and copies of free pamphlets on many related subjects including:
  - Reducing your risk of heart attack.
  - Controlling high blood pressure.
  - Eating to keep your heart healthy.
  - How to stop smoking.
  - Exercising for good health.

SOME WORDS OF CAUTION

- If you have diabetes, gout, or a family history of heart disease, your real risk of developing heart disease will be greater than indicated by your RISKO score. If your score is high and you have one or more of these additional problems, you should give particular attention to reducing your risk.

- If you are a woman under 45 years or a man under 35 years of age, your RISKO score represents an upper limit on your real risk of developing heart disease. In this case, your real risk is probably lower than indicated by your score.
- Using your weight category to estimate your systolic blood pressure or your blood cholesterol level makes your RISKO score less accurate.
- Your score will tend to overestimate your risk if your actual values on these two important factors are average for someone of your height and weight.
- Your score will underestimate your risk if your actual blood pressure or cholesterol level is above average for someone of your height or weight.

UNDERSTANDING HEART DISEASE

In the United States it is estimated that close to 550,000 people die each year from coronary heart disease. Coronary artery disease is the most common type of heart disease and the leading cause of death in the United States and many other countries.

Coronary heart disease is the result of coronary atherosclerosis. Coronary atherosclerosis is the name of the process by which an accumulation of fatty deposits leads to a thickening and narrowing of the inner walls of the arteries that carry oxygenated blood and nutrients to the heart muscle. The effect is similar to that of a water pipe clogged by deposits.

The resulting restriction of the blood supply to the heart muscle can cause injury to the muscle as well as angina (chest pain). If the restriction of the blood supply is severe or if it continues over a period of time, the heart muscle cells fed by the restricted artery suffer irreversible injury and die. This is known as a myocardial infarction or heart attack.

Scientists have identified a number of factors which are linked with an increased likelihood or risk of developing coronary heart disease. Some of these risk factors, like aging, being male, or having a family history of heart disease, are unavoidable. However, many other significant risk factors, including all of the factors used to determine your RISKO score, can be changed to reduce the likelihood of developing heart disease.

Cholesterol in bloodstream

Blood vessel

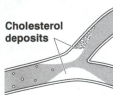

Blood

Cholesterol deposits

APPRAISING YOUR RISK

- The RISKO heart hazard appraisal is an indicator of risk for adults who do not currently show evidence of heart disease. However, if you already have heart disease, it is very important that you work with your doctor in reducing your risk.
- The original concept of RISKO was developed by the Michigan Heart Association. It has been further developed by the American Heart Association with the assistance of Drs. John and Sonja McKinlay in Boston. It is based on Framingham, Stanford, and Chicago heart disease studies. The format of RISKO was tested and refined by Dr. Robert M. Chamberlain and Dr. Armin Weinberg of the National Heart Center at the Baylor College of Medicine in Houston, Texas.

What Can I Do Now?

Are you physically fit right now? Are your muscles as toned as you want them to be? Are you comfortable with your weight? Do you know what your measurements are today? Do you have any idea what your aerobic fitness level is? Be sure you fill out, on a regular basis, the Body Measurement Chart, Modified Step Test Checklist, and Flexibility Checklist that follow. Complete the Student Health History Form located in Appendix A and give it to your instructor.

What Condition Are You in Now?

What condition are you in now? You may look pretty good in the mirror, but are you aerobically fit? Perhaps you are, but maybe you're carrying a few extra pounds that you would like to shed. It is important to evaluate your current fitness level so that you (1) are aware of your current status, and (2) can measure your progress. There is nothing better than seeing progress to help you stick with and enjoy a regular exercise program.

When you begin an exercise program, the initial discomforts of fatigue, possible muscle soreness, dry mouth, and labored breathing seem discouraging. Try to remember there is no such thing as instant fitness—the benefits take about 6 to 12 weeks to appear. You must commit yourself to your exercise program. If you are not committed and persistent, you may drop out before the results are apparent. Keeping a progress chart will help you visualize your progress and stay with your exercise program.

There is an easy way to visualize your progress. Gains, even small ones, can be measured right from the start. When you begin a new exercise program, take a good look at yourself in the mirror and assess your body appearance, so that you can observe your improved appearance and become aware of your progress. Becoming aware of your progress is a self-motivator and will help you stick to your exercise program. The three areas in which you can easily perform a self-assessment are personal measurements, aerobic capacity, and flexibility.

Closely examine your body in a mirror before beginning an exercise program, so that you can measure your progress.

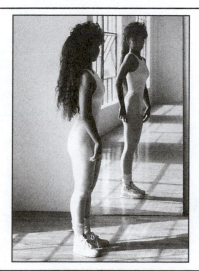

Body Measurement					
Directions: Weigh yourself and take your body measurements throughout the semester at the intervals listed below; record the results on the chart and monitor your progress.					
	Before Week 1	After Week 4	After Week 8	After Week 12	After Week 16
Weight					
Upper arm (measure halfway between the shoulder joint and the elbow)					
Chest					
Waist					
Hips (measure 7 in. below the waist)					
Upper thigh (measure halfway between the hip joint and the knee)					
Calf					

Assessing Your Personal Measurements

It is sometimes awkward to take your own measurements. Try to find a trusted friend to help you complete the above chart. Or, take your own measurements. Fill out the chart before you begin your aqua aerobics exercise program, again 4 weeks into the program, and again after 8, 12, and 16 weeks of exercising. If you keep the chart accurate, you will be able to compare your body measurements throughout the semester. You will be amazed at your progress!

A friend can help take your measurements.

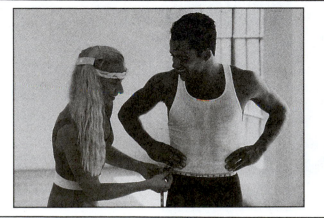

Testing Your Aerobic Capacity

To test your current aerobic fitness level, perform the modified step test that follows. This test is easy to execute and will allow you to assess your personal progress throughout the semester if you repeat it on the same schedule as the body measurement chart.

Modified Step Test

You need a stopwatch, an eight-inch step (such as those in the average staircase), and a chair to complete this test.

Directions: Step up and down, alternating feet, for three minutes at a rate of approximately one complete sequence every two seconds. Stop at exactly three minutes, and immediately sit in a chair. After one minute of rest, take your pulse for 30 seconds, and multiply it by two to obtain your one-minute pulse recovery score. Compare your score to the chart on the following page to find your starting aerobic condition.

Assessing Your Modified Step Test Score

If you have been sedentary, your score will most likely be near 100 or slightly above, regardless of your age. If you are exceptionally fit, your score will be below that of someone your age who is less fit.

If your score on the modified step test is well below 100, and it falls within the very high or high rating, you already have a high cardiovascular/cardiorespiratory endurance level. Keep up the good work!

If your score is within the moderate or low rating, there is room for improvement in your cardiovascular/cardiorespiratory endurance level.

If your score falls within the very low rating, a regular aerobic program will make a big difference in your cardiovascular/cardiorespiratory endurance level.

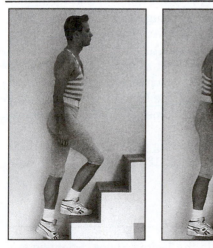

a. Modified step test   b.

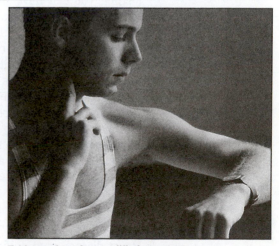

Taking pulse after modified step test

Training Heart Rates
Aerobic fitness rating according to heartbeats per minute

Age	Very High	High	Moderate	Low	Very Low
Female					
10-19	Below 82	82-91	92-97	98-102	Above 102
20-29	Below 83	83-87	88-93	94-98	Above 98
30-39	Below 83	82-89	90-95	96-98	Above 98
40-49	Below 83	82-87	88-97	98-102	Above 102
Over 50	Below 86	86-93	94-99	100-104	Above 104
Male					
10-19	Below 72	72-77	78-83	84-88	Above 88
20-29	Below 72	72-79	80-85	86-93	Above 93
30-39	Below 76	76-81	82-87	88-93	Above 93
40-49	Below 78	78-83	84-89	90-94	Above 94
Over 50	Below 80	80-85	86-91	92-95	Above 95

	Before Week 1	After Week 4	After Week 8	After Week 12	After Week 16
Your Score:					

Testing Your General Flexibility

Flexibility is specific to a joint or a combination of joints. Through extensive testing, you can have the flexibility in every joint evaluated and identified. However, you can measure general flexibility by using the Sit and Reach Test. To perform this test, you need a sit and reach box. Ask your instructor where you can find one or you can build one yourself (see Appendix G).

To do the test, sit with the soles of your feet flat against the sit and reach box. Keeping your knees straight but not locked, reach forward with your arms fully extended, palms down, fingers straight, and one hand on top of the other. Hold this position for three seconds. Repeat three times and use the best score (the longest stretch).

Compare your score to the chart on the following page to assess your flexibility. Repeat this test at the end of weeks 4, 8, 12, and 16 to follow your progress in increasing flexibility.

Your Heart

Heart disease is at epidemic proportions in the United States. Scientific evidence indicates that regular cardiovascular exercise strengthens the heart mus-

Sit and Reach Flexibility Test*

	17-19	20-29	30-39	40-49	50-59	60-65
			Age			
			Reach (in centimeters)			
Males						
Excellent	>48	>45	>45	>43	>42	>41
Good	37-48	37-44	34-44	32-42	31-41	29-40
Minimum	26-36	25-35	25-33	22-31	19-30	18-28
Below Minimum	15-25	15-24	14-23	11-21	8-18	6-17
Poor	<14	<14	<12	<10	<7	<5
Females						
Excellent	>43	>41	>38	>35	>32	>28
Good	39-42	38-40	35-37	32-34	28-31	25-27
Minimum	37-39	34-37	31-34	28-30	23-26	21-24
Below Minimum	34-36	31-33	28-30	24-27	19-22	18-20
Poor	<33	<30	<27	<23	<17	<16

*Note: Footline set at 25 centimeters.

	Before Week 1	After Week 4	After Week 8	After Week 12	After Week 16
Your Score:					

Sit and reach test

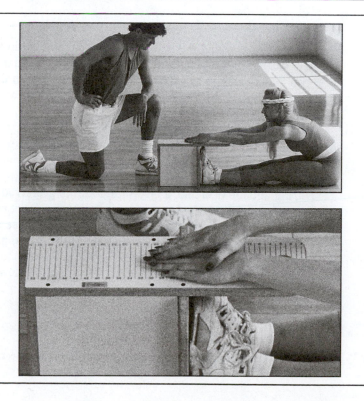

cle and reduces the risk of cardiovascular problems. According to R.S. Paffenbarger and R.T. Hyde, "Evidence mounts that the relationship between exercise and good health is more than circumstantial. If some questions are not yet answered, they are far less important than those that have been."*

Through exercise overload, the heart muscle becomes more fit and is able to work more efficiently and effectively. The more fit the heart is, the more oxygen-carrying blood can be pumped to the body with each contraction of the heart. Thus, a fit heart does not need to work as hard or beat as frequently as a less-fit heart. In discussing cardiovascular fitness and efficiency, you need to be aware of your resting heart rate, your target heart rate, and your recovery heart rate.

Resting Heart Rate

Resting heart rate refers to the number of times your heart beats per minute upon waking or when you have been sitting or resting for approximately 10 minutes. The best time to take your resting heart rate is when you first wake up and are still lying down. To obtain the most accurate reading, take your pulse for 60 seconds on three consecutive mornings, and then average the three numbers. A person who exercises regularly may have a lower resting heart rate than a person who is sedentary. An average resting heart rate for adults is approximately 72 beats per minute. If you discover that your resting heart rate has decreased after several months of participation in an aerobic exercise, it is an indication that your fitness level has improved. That's an improvement you would like to see!

Taking Your Pulse

For most people, taking the pulse is easiest at the carotid artery. The carotid pulse is located in the groove of the neck, next to the Adam's apple. Use your first two fingers and press lightly on the carotid artery on the same side of the body as the hand you are using (be careful not to press too hard). You will feel your pulse beating.

Another place to take your pulse is at the radial artery (on the thumb side of your wrist, palm up). When taking your pulse, be sure to use the first two or three fingers, not the thumb. The thumb has a pulse of its own and therefore could cause an inaccurate reading.

During aquatic exercise, a 6-second count is preferred due to the water's cooling effect on the body. In this environment the heart rate may drop more quickly than during land-based exercising, where a 10-second pulse count is most often recommended. When taking your pulse, it is important that you continue to move slowly through the water so that proper blood flow is maintained. Stopping suddenly after exercising can alter the blood flow through the body, which can lead to dizziness or mild nausea.

*R.S. Paffenbarger and R.T. Hyde, "Exercise as Protection against Heart Attack," *New England Journal of Medicine* 301 (1980), p. 1026.

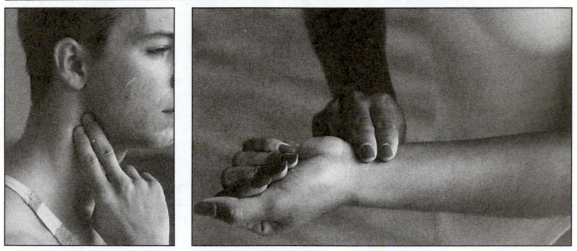

Pulse at the carotid artery   **Pulse at the radial artery**

Checklist: Taking Your Pulse

1. With your index and middle fingers (not your thumb) you can find your pulse in the carotid artery very easily: Place your fingers on your Adam's apple. Gently slide your fingers toward the outside of the neck, into the natural "notch" on the side of your neck. By pressing lightly, you can feel the pulse at the carotid artery.

2. You can find your radial pulse by placing your fingers lightly on the inside of your wrist. To do this, rotate one arm in so the palm of your hand is facing you. Then place the fingers of the opposite hand just above your wrist on the thumb side and just inside the arm bone (the radius). You will feel the radial pulse.

3. While at rest, practice counting the number of pulse beats for one minute by:
   a. Counting your pulse for 15 seconds and multiplying by 4.
   b. Counting your pulse for 10 seconds and multiplying by 6.
   c. Counting your pulse for 6 seconds and multiplying by 10.

Target Heart Rate

Target heart rate (THR) is the heart rate level you must work toward to gain enough benefits from exercising to improve cardiovascular fitness. There are several methods established for calculating target heart rate; two accepted formulas will be described here. Use both formulas, compare the two results, and choose the level where you will work. (You may choose an average of the two results.)

You need first to determine the intensity level at which you would like to work. A person who has been sedentary for a long time may want to begin an exercise regimen at the 50 percent level and work up gradually to 70 percent. It is generally accepted that for most people, 70 percent is a good level at which to work. Athletes and highly fit individuals may work at 90 percent.

In accordance with the exercise guidelines set forth by the American College of Sports Medicine, one should use percentages associated with low, average, or high cardiorespiratory levels of fitness:*

Low fitness	60 to 65 percent heart rate reserve
Average fitness	70 to 80 percent heart rate reserve
High fitness	80 to 90 percent heart rate reserve

Second, you must determine your resting heart rate. Once you determine your intensity level and your resting heart rate, proceed with the following formulas and techniques to find your exercise target heart rate range. The target heart rate range is the lower and upper heart rate levels you must achieve (and stay between) during exercise to gain an aerobic benefit from your exercise period.

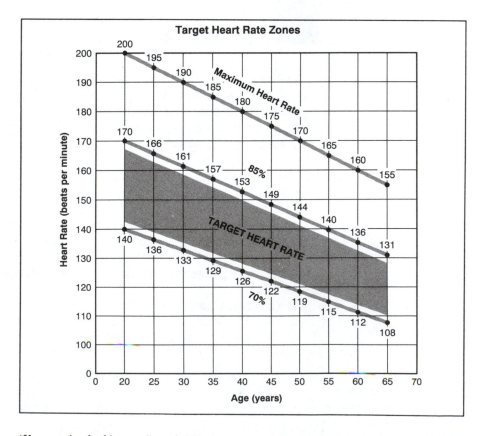

*If you are involved in a cardiac rehabilitation program, it is strongly advised to begin at a 50 to 55 percent heart rate reserve.

The Karvonen Method

The formula for the Karvonen method of determining the target heart rate is as follows:

THR = INTENSITY x (MHR – RHR) + RHR, where
THR = Target heart rate,
MHR = Maximum heart rate,
RHR = Resting heart rate, and
THR = 60% to 90% x (MHR – RHR) + RHR

To help you better understand the Karvonen formula, an example follows for a 20-year-old person working at 70 percent intensity with an 80 beats-per-minute resting heart rate:

MHR = 220 minus age
        220 – 20
MHR = 200

To determine the target heart rate at 70 percent (lower end of the target heart rate range):

THR = .70 x (MHR – RHR) + RHR
     = .70 x (200 – 80) + 80
     = .70 x (120) + 80
     = 84 + 80
THR = 164

To determine the target heart rate at 85 percent (upper end of target heart rate range):

THR = .85 x (MHR – RHR) + RHR
     = .85 x (200 – 80) + 80
     = .85 x (120) + 80
     = 102 + 80
THR = 182

Divide the target heart rate by 10 at the lower and upper ends of the range to get the number you need for a 6-second pulse count:

164 ÷ 10 = 16.4
182 ÷ 10 = 18.2

To work at the 70 percent level of intensity, this 20-year-old would strive to work at 16 pulse beats during a 6-second count and not exceed 18 beats, because that represents an 85 percent intensity. (If you are an athlete, use 90 percent as the upper limit.)

The American College of Sports Medicine Method

The American College of Sports Medicine recommends a simpler formula. Just subtract your age from 220, multiply by the desired intensity of your workout level, and divide the answer by 10 for a 6-second pulse beat estimate. It is recommended that your working target heart rate be 65 to 85 percent of your maximum heart rate.

The following example is again for a 20-year-old working at the 70 percent level:

220 − 20	=	200	Maximum heart rate
200 x .7	=	140	Target heart rate (THR)
140 + 10	=	14	Number of pulse beats in a 6-second period

To find the upper end of the range, multiply by 85 percent (90 percent if you are an athlete):

220 − 20	=	200
200 x .85	=	170
170 + 10	=	17

To work at the desired level of intensity, this 20-year-old would consider the results of both formulas and strive for 14 to 18 pulse beats during a 6-second count.

Be careful not to work over your target heart rate for more than a few seconds. You will not get into shape any faster; actually, working over your target heart rate may fatigue you faster, cause you discomfort, and even be unhealthy for you. Use common sense to check your exertion: if you are feeling extreme fatigue, you are probably overworking yourself.

Perceived Exertion Rating Scale

In addition to the target heart rate method of determining the desired level of exercise, the perceived exertion rating scale, developed by Swedish physiologist Gunnar Borg, provides an exerciser with a subjective description of how intensely he/she is working out. Your own estimate of how much effort it takes to perform a given task is called *perceived exertion* and can be a reliable guide to determining the intensity of the cardiovascular output during your workout. In other words, perceived exertion involves monitoring how you feel when exercising and using that to guide your cardiovascular workout. In fact, recent studies indicate that people who learn to listen to their bodies and go by their rate of perceived exertion work as hard, if not more efficiently, as those who get "hung up on the numbers." The perceived exertion rating scale ranges from 6 to 20. Due to the variables that can affect a workout, such as water temperature, weather (if you're outdoors), mood, and how you are feeling physically on that given day, the rate of perceived exertion is being used as a monitoring tool in many aquatic exercise programs.

The chart on the following page is adapted from the Borg scale. Select a number within the range listed that best describes your level of exertion while exercising, and multiply that number by 10. The resulting product may be close to your working heart rate.

Rating Scale of Perceived Exertion	
6	Very, very light
8	Very light
10	Light
12	Moderate
14	Somewhat hard
16	Hard
18	Very hard
20	Very, very hard

Research has indicated that rate of perceived exertion (RPE) monitoring generally corresponds to heart rate monitoring. An individual who describes his/her workout as "very light," number 8 on the RPE scale, is usually exercising at the 60 percent level. One that defines his/her workout to be "very hard," number 18 on the RPE scale, is usually working out between 80 to 90 percent. Check this system out for yourself and see if you find an accurate correlation between the RPE scale and target heart rate monitoring.

In addition to the fact that RPE is an accurate measurement for aquatic exercisers due to the circumstances previously described, using this scale helps you focus on how you are feeling during your workout rather than on counting your pulse rate. You can ask yourself the following questions while exercising:

- Is my breathing rhythmic or quick and shallow while I'm working out? If your breathing is rhythmic, then you are relaxed and breathing properly. If your breathing is quick and shallow, then you may be exhibiting stress while exercising. You need to relax and concentrate on breathing more rhythmically. Rhythmic, steady breathing is necessary to assist your body in adapting to the stress of exercise and to permit a good flow of oxygen and carbon dioxide exchange in your bloodstream.
- Am I completing all of my movements, or am I rushing through them? To get the most out of exercising you should complete all of your movements, even if it means you are moving more slowly than your classmates.
- Is this hard for me? Can I work harder?
- How am I feeling while exercising?

Another type of perceived exertion is a method that has been commonly called the "talk test." This method of identifying exercise intensity means that you should be able to talk or sing while executing your aqua aerobics endurance movements.

Monitoring Your Heart Rate

Monitoring your heart rate during exercise is extremely important, to make sure that you are exercising at an intensity high enough to reach your target heart rate but not so high that you exceed your target heart rate by too much. Take your pulse before class, twice during the aqua aerobics portion of class, and once during the cool-down phase of class. Your instructor will most likely lead the group, but if not, monitor your heart rate yourself. You need to make sure that you are working within your appropriate target heart rate zone. If, when checking your pulse, you discover you are working at too high a level, adjust your movements to reduce the intensity of the workout. To reduce the intensity of exercise, make your arm movements smaller and weaker, don't lift your legs as high as you did previously, and slow your movements down a little. On the other hand, if you find you are not working as high as your target heart rate, increase your workload by making larger movements or exerting more power while resisting the water, and perhaps by moving a little faster. It is important to note that to improve cardiovascular fitness you must work within the 50 to 85 percent target heart rate range. However, remember the only way to exercise safely is to progress gradually to these levels.

Warning About Taking Heart Rate During Aqua Aerobics

As you just read, monitoring your heart rate during aerobic exercise is important. It is also important to check your recovery heart rate following exercise. However, a recent position paper by the American College of Sports Medicine recommends using as a measurement of exercise intensity not only target heart rate but also perceived exertion.

Another concern when using the target heart rate monitoring system in water activities is that many factors commonly associated with water exercising will increase the heart rate while not increasing the use of oxygen in the body. The factors that can cause an increase in heart rate are:

- *Shallow water*—Performing aqua aerobics in shallow water will increase your heart rate because the shallower the water, the more impact you will experience. Shallow water offers less resistance and allows you to perform movements faster, which will increase your heart rate faster than slower movements will. In addition, shallow water exposes the body more to the air; if the air is much warmer than the water, core temperature will increase. As core temperature increases, more blood flows to the body's periphery in order to cool off the body. This action lowers cardiac return, causing heart rate to increase in order to maintain cardiac output. It is recommended that the air temperature be kept three degrees warmer than the water in indoor pools.

- *Hot air*—When you exercise in an environment with high air temperature, your heart rate will increase just to help cool down your body.

- *Bathing cap*—Performing water exercises with a rubber bathing cap on does not allow the body to dissipate heat through the head. Therefore, your core body temperature will increase since your body can't eliminate heat as rapidly as it usually can, and your heart rate will increase to help cool down your body.

- *Very warm water*—Working out in water that is 88° to 90° will increase your heart rate due to your body's reduced ability to dissipate the heat created during exercising. (However, since most public pools are kept between 78° and 84°, this would not be a concern for many exercisers.)

- *Arms overhead*—Performing aquatic exercises with your arms overhead will raise your heart rate because your arms are up. Also, having your arms out of the water and exposed to the air, which may be warmer than the water, could cause your heart rate to rise.

Other Factors Affecting Heart Rate Responses

Other factors that can increase or decrease heart rate include:

- *Ambient air temperature*—The temperature of the air will have an effect on your heart rate response. As described above, hot air will cause your heart rate to increase, to help cool down your body. When the body surface is exposed to cool air the core temperature of the body will decrease, thus causing a lower heart rate response. Persons exercising outdoors or in pools where the air temperature is lower than the water temperature should be careful to perform most of their arm movements underwater. Exposing the arms to cooler air will cause the exercise heart rate to decrease as the body attempts to keep the core temperature up. Again, in this situation it is important to use the perceived exertion rating scale to monitor the exercise exertion level so that you can have another indicator of exercise.

- *Medication*—Certain medications, such as beta blockers taken for various heart conditions, will cause the heart rate to decrease. An individual using such medication will have a false reading if he/she is evaluating his/her exercise level by target heart rate and is not using the perceived exertion method. Other types of medications may speed up the heart rate—again, an individual using the target heart rate method would have a false reading as to the effectiveness of his/her exercising.

- *Caffeine*—Caffeine will increase heart rate. Drinking coffee or caffeinated sodas or taking drugs containing caffeine before class may increase the heart rate and give you a false reading.

- *Smoking*—Cigarettes will increase the heart rate. Smoking before class is not advisable as it will increase your heart rate and yield an inaccurate indication of your exercising level.

- *Anxiety*—Anxiety usually speeds up the heart rate. An anxious exerciser may have a false reading when using the target heart rate method to measure the effectiveness of his/her exercising.

The aforementioned reasons are just some examples to support the theory for using the perceived exertion rating scale during aqua aerobics classes. However, it should be noted that medication, caffeine, smoking, and anxiety can also alter a person's personal perception of his/her exercise exertion. The perceived exertion scale relies on an individual's perceptions. External factors such as those just described could cause that evaluation to be somewhat inaccurate. The perceived exertion rating scale is a good indicator of exercise intensity, but it is not infallible.

When monitoring your own heart rate during an exercise session, be aware of the elements just listed that contribute to an increase or decrease in heart rate. It is a good idea to follow the latest suggestion made by the American

College of Sports Medicine and use the perceived exertion method of monitoring your heart rate in conjunction with the target heart rate method.*

Recovery Heart Rate

Your recovery heart rate is how quickly your pulse returns to normal after a workout involving aerobic activity such as aquatic exercise. The more aerobically conditioned you are, the faster your heart rate will return to normal (or recover). Take your pulse two to five minutes after exercising. Your heart rate should recover to close to normal and be below 100 beats per minute five minutes after your class has ended.

Normally, a cool-down is led by your instructor during the last 10 minutes of class to guide your body to return to its pre-exercise heart rate. If you do not perform a proper cool-down your body could go into a mild type of shock recovery, which might leave you feeling light-headed, dizzy, and possibly even mildly nauseous.

Caution

Do not leave class until you have participated in the cool-down. You could end up fainting due to your body's lack of ability to readjust your circulation from the exercising phase to the recovery phase.

Evaluating Your Recovery Heart Rate

Take your pulse two to five minutes after exercising.

If you have a decrease from your target heart rate of . . .	Then your recovery heart rate is . . .
60 beats per minute	Super
50 beats per minute	Excellent
40 beats per minute	Good
30 beats per minute	Acceptable

After several months of consistently working out aerobically, you may notice that your heart rate recovers faster and is lower than before you began your aquatic exercise regimen. Your heart rate should return to its pre-exercise level within 10 minutes after your aquatic exercise class ends. If it doesn't, you may have overexerted yourself during the aerobics portion of the class. Reduce the intensity of your workout during the next class, and monitor the length of time

*"The Recommended Quantity and Quality of Exercise for Developing and Maintaining Cardiorespiratory and Muscular Fitness in Healthy Adults," *Medicine and Science in Sports and Exercise*, April 1990.

it takes for your heart rate to return to normal. If your heart rate does not return to its pre-exercise level within 10 minutes following that class, consult your physician or your instructor.

Principles of Conditioning

The principles of conditioning include frequency of exercise, intensity of exercise, duration of exercise, and the rate of progression of training.

Frequency of Exercise

Frequency of exercise refers to how often you exercise per week. To obtain maximum benefits from working out, you should participate in aqua aerobics or a combination of other aerobic-type activities three to five times a week. The aerobic portion of class should last at least 20 minutes and should not exceed 60 minutes per class period. If you exercise only once a week, you will not improve your fitness level and will probably be sore after exercising because of the stress you have placed on unconditioned muscles. But by the same token, exercising every day is not necessary. Studies have shown that people who rest at least one day a week have fewer injuries than those who exercise daily. Similarly, exercising three to five times a week appears to be as beneficial as exercising six or seven days a week. The body needs time to rest and recuperate so that you can avoid straining muscles. An occasional day off is of great value in developing and maintaining fitness, both physically and psychologically.

Intensity of Exercise

Intensity of exercise refers to how hard you work when exercising. Once you have identified your target heart rate and are familiar with the perceived exertion rating system, you should continually monitor the intensity at which you are working. Working too hard is ineffective, and can make you sore or result in an injury. The key is to find the optimal level of intensity for your body that will help you meet your goals.

Duration of Exercise

Duration of exercise refers to how long you work out at one time. The duration of an exercise session depends on the component of fitness you are trying to develop. You must spend time on each component of fitness as well as on each muscle group. Duration and frequency of activity are primary concerns of your exercise program in order to improve your health and fitness level; decrease body fat; lose or maintain body weight; enhance the cardiovascular system; and increase muscular strength, muscular endurance, and flexibility. For the cardiovascular component, you must do a minimum of 20 continuous minutes of concentrated effort in your target heart rate zone. Strength and endurance are developed as you overload the muscles gradually and increase the number of repetitions and sets of work on each muscle group. As set forth by the American College of Sports Medicine (ACSM), exercising three to five times per week for 20 to 60 minutes is sufficient to gain notable improvements in your

Checklist: Semester Progress

It is valuable to identify your progress throughout the semester. Complete the following for each week listed.

	Before Week 1	After Week 4	After Week 8	After Week 12	After Week 16
Weight					
Waist measurement					
Upper arm measurement (around biceps/ triceps muscle area), right arm					
Upper arm measurement, left arm					
Thigh measurement (3" below crotch)					
Hips measurement (7" below the waist)					
Resting heart rate					
Target heart rate					
Sit and reach flexibility					
Modified step test					
Maximum number of push-ups					
Number of curl-ups in 1 minute					

health and fitness levels. A 50- to 60-minute aqua aerobic class that meets three to five times per week and follows the ACSM guidelines will provide you with a good duration of exercise for meeting most of your goals.

Rate of Progression of Training

The statement "No pain, no gain" makes no sense. A gradual increase in your workload by application of the overload principle is both safe and effective. Trying to do too much too soon will pave the way to exhaustion and may cause injury and discourage you from being consistent with your exercise program. As set forth by the American College of Sports Medicine's guidelines for an exercise program, the rate of progression is as follows:

- *Initial conditioning*—Four to six weeks, depending on your current fitness level and adaptation to your workout program.

- *Improvement conditioning*—Twelve to 20 weeks; intensity is increased to 50 to 85 percent of your cardiovascular functional capacity. Refer to the section on target heart rate to determine your personal level.

- *Maintenance conditioning*—After the first six months of training, you will want to review your program objectives and evaluate your progress.

Summary

1. Research has established that regular, vigorous exercise is beneficial to the human body in many ways. The benefits are as follows:
   - An individual feels good after exercising aerobically.
   - Stress and tension in the body are reduced.
   - Risk of coronary heart disease is lowered.
   - Muscle fibers perform more efficiently.
   - Bones become denser, and therefore are strengthened.
   - Weight control is easier because all forms of aerobic exercise will raise your metabolic rate and allow you to burn more calories for several hours following your workout.
   - The heart muscle becomes stronger and more efficient.

2. The five components of fitness are
   - Cardiorespiratory endurance and cardiovascular efficiency.
   - Muscular strength.
   - Muscular endurance.
   - Flexibility.
   - Body composition.

3. The body is composed of both lean body mass and fat. The amount of fat on the body is measured by underwater weighing, electrical impedance, skinfold calipers, or circumferential measurements. It is recommended that fat as a component of the body should not exceed 18 percent for men and 22 percent for women.

4. Factors known to increase the risks of cardiovascular disease are
   - A family history of heart disease.
   - High blood pressure.
   - Cigarette smoking.
   - Being overweight.
   - High levels of triglycerides and cholesterol in the blood.
   - Diabetes.
   - Stress.
   - Physical inactivity.

5. Regularly fill out the body measurement chart so that you can visualize your results.

6. Complete the modified step test several times throughout the semester to evaluate your aerobic fitness level. Watch your improvement!

7. Be sure to perform the sit and reach test regularly to see your progress.

8. Remember, there is no such thing as instant fitness. It takes 6 to 12 weeks of consistent participation in an aqua aerobics class before you will see results.

9. To understand your cardiovascular fitness and efficiency, you must be aware of and know how to calculate your:
   - Resting heart rate.
   - Target heart rate.
   - Maximum heart rate.
   - Recovery heart rate.

10. Another method for evaluating the effectiveness of your workout is to use the perceived exertion rating scale.

11. You can take your pulse easily by using the carotid or the radial pulse.

12. The "talk test" refers to one's ability to talk or sing while performing aqua aerobics movements.

13. The minimum number of times you need to exercise in order to achieve aerobic benefits is three sessions per week:
    - For greater aerobic benefit, exercise five times per week.
    - Participating in a 50- to 60-minute aqua aerobics class three to five times per week will help you meet most of your fitness goals.

14. To get the proper duration of exercise:
    - You must increase the sets and repetitions of exercise for each muscle group to improve the strength component of fitness.
    - You must do a minimum of 20 continuous minutes of concentrated effort in your target heart rate zone for the cardiovascular component. Thirty continuous minutes of concentrated effort in your target heart rate zone will yield greater benefits to your cardiovascular system.

15. Fill out the Checklist in this chapter entitled "Semester Progress" at the appropriate times throughout your course to get an overall view of your progress.

16. Now you are on the road to improving your fitness and feeling better. Congratulations!

CHAPTER 3

Anatomy, Body Types, and Body Alignment

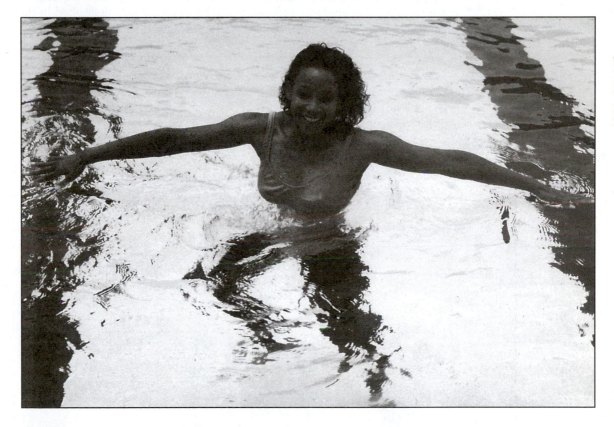

Outline

Anatomy
Checklist: Bones and Muscles
Somatotypes or Body Types
Body Alignment
Summary

Anatomy

While you are working out in your aqua aerobics class, your instructor may make reference to muscles you are using. For this reason and the fact that you are now involved in a regular exercise program and are interested in your body, you should know a little about basic anatomy.

Anatomy is described as the structural makeup of the human body. For your purposes, as an exercise enthusiast, the main bones of the body and the main muscles that apply to exercising will be depicted and described in this chapter.

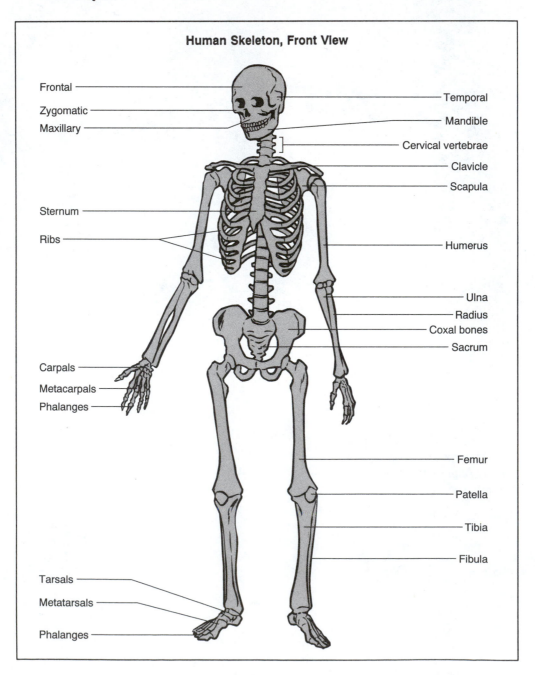

Human Skeleton, Front View

Frontal — Temporal
Zygomatic — Mandible
Maxillary — Cervical vertebrae
— Clavicle
— Scapula
Sternum — Humerus
Ribs —
— Ulna
— Radius
— Coxal bones
— Sacrum
Carpals —
Metacarpals —
Phalanges —
— Femur
— Patella
— Tibia
— Fibula
Tarsals —
Metatarsals —
Phalanges —

Human Skeleton, Back View

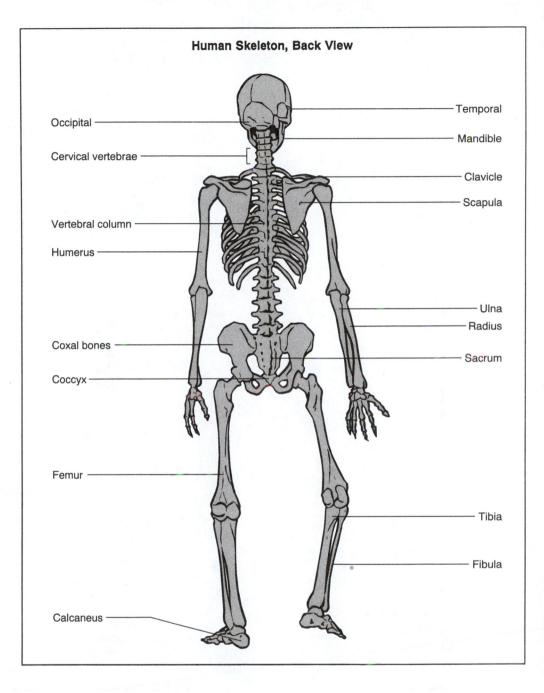

Occipital

Cervical vertebrae

Vertebral column

Humerus

Coxal bones

Coccyx

Femur

Calcaneus

Temporal

Mandible

Clavicle

Scapula

Ulna

Radius

Sacrum

Tibia

Fibula

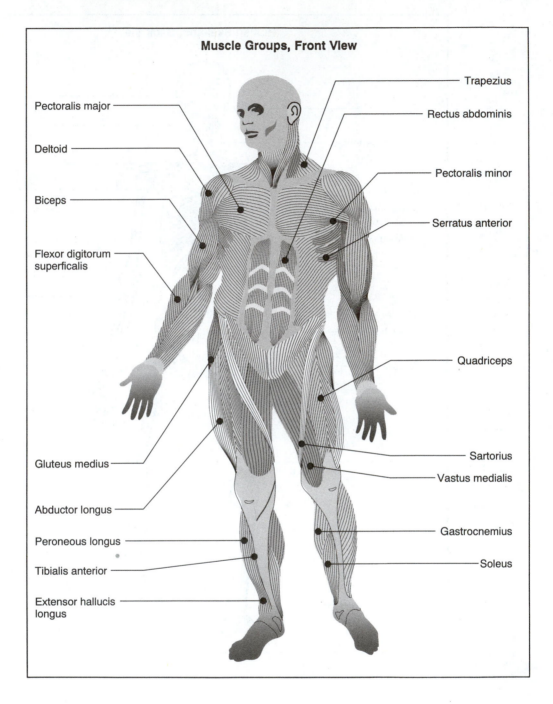

Muscle Groups, Front View

Trapezius

Rectus abdominis

Pectoralis minor

Serratus anterior

Quadriceps

Sartorius

Vastus medialis

Gastrocnemius

Soleus

Pectoralis major

Deltoid

Biceps

Flexor digitorum superficalis

Gluteus medius

Abductor longus

Peroneous longus

Tibialis anterior

Extensor hallucis longus

Muscle Groups, Back View

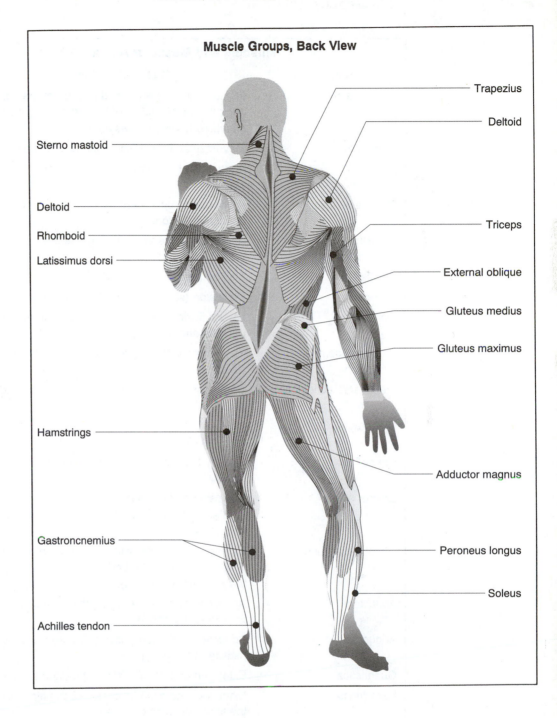

Sterno mastoid

Deltoid

Rhomboid

Latissimus dorsi

Hamstrings

Gastroncnemius

Achilles tendon

Trapezius

Deltoid

Triceps

External oblique

Gluteus medius

Gluteus maximus

Adductor magnus

Peroneus longus

Soleus

Muscles and Muscular Action

Muscle	Muscular Action
Sternocleidomastoid	Flexion, lateral flexion, and rotation of the head and neck (forward bending of the head, bringing ear to shoulder, looking sideways).
Trapezius	Movements of the scapula (shoulder blades).
Deltoid	Abduction of the arms (raising the arms from the sides).
Pectoralis major	Forward and downward movements of the arm and horizontal flexion.
Latissimus dorsi	Adduction of the arms (pulling the arms down from the sides).
Biceps	Flexion (bending) of the elbow.
Triceps	Extension (straightening) of the elbow.
Oblique	Lateral flexion and rotation of the trunk (bending to the side and twisting).
Rectus abdominis	Flexion of the trunk (bending forward from the waist).
Transverse abdominis	Compression of the abdomen (pulling the abdomen in).
Diaphragm	Initiates breathing by increasing the size of the chest cavity.
Hip flexor	Flexion of the hip joint (bringing the leg toward the head).
Erector spinae	Extension and hyperextension of the spine (straightening up from the waist and bending backwards).
Gluteus maximus	Extension and hyperextension of the hip (bringing the leg up toward the body in the rear, and behind the body from the front).
Abductors	Abduction of the leg (moving the leg away from the midline to the body).
Adductors	Adduction of the leg (moving the leg toward the midline of the body).
Quadriceps	Extension of the knee (straightening the knee).
Hamstrings	Extension and hyperextension of the hip; flexion of the knee (bending the knee).
Gastrocnemius	Plantar flexion of the foot at the ankle (pointing the foot).
Soleus	Plantar flexion of the foot at the ankle (pointing the foot).
Tibialis anterior	Flexing (lifting) the front of the foot up while the heel is down.

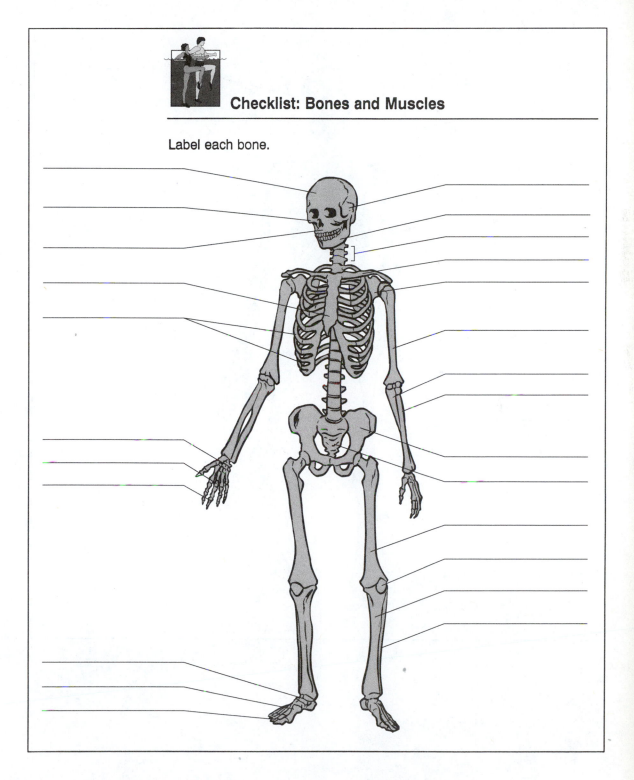

Checklist: Bones and Muscles

Label each bone.

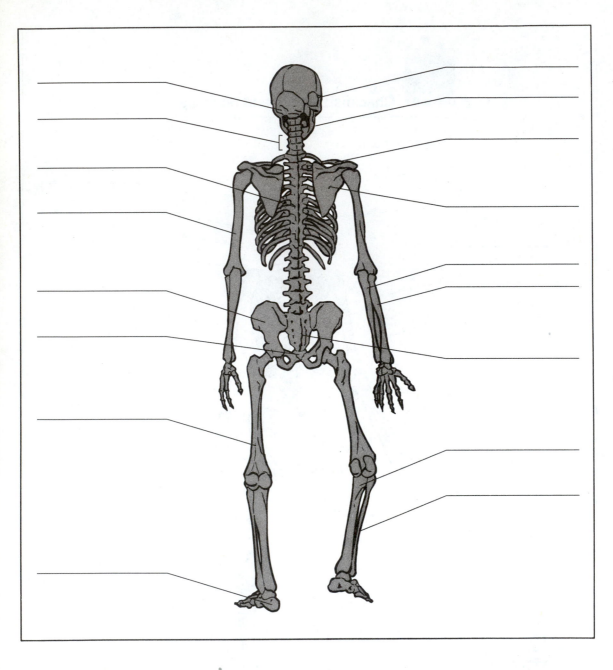

Label each muscle.

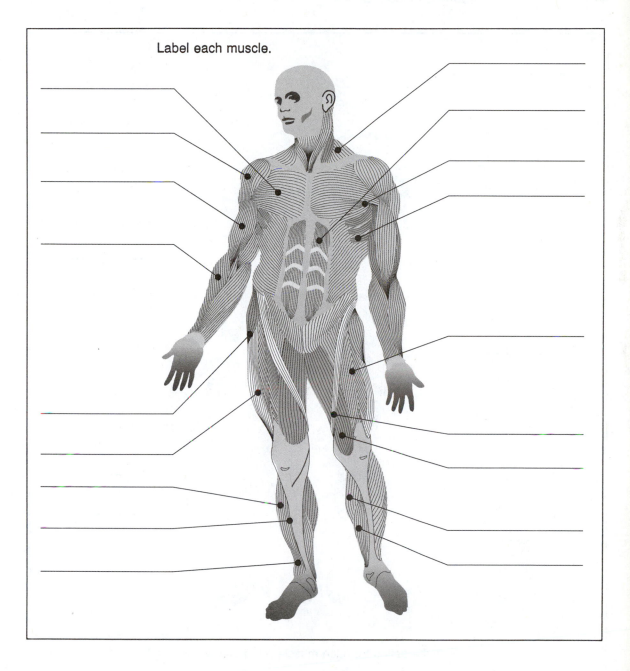

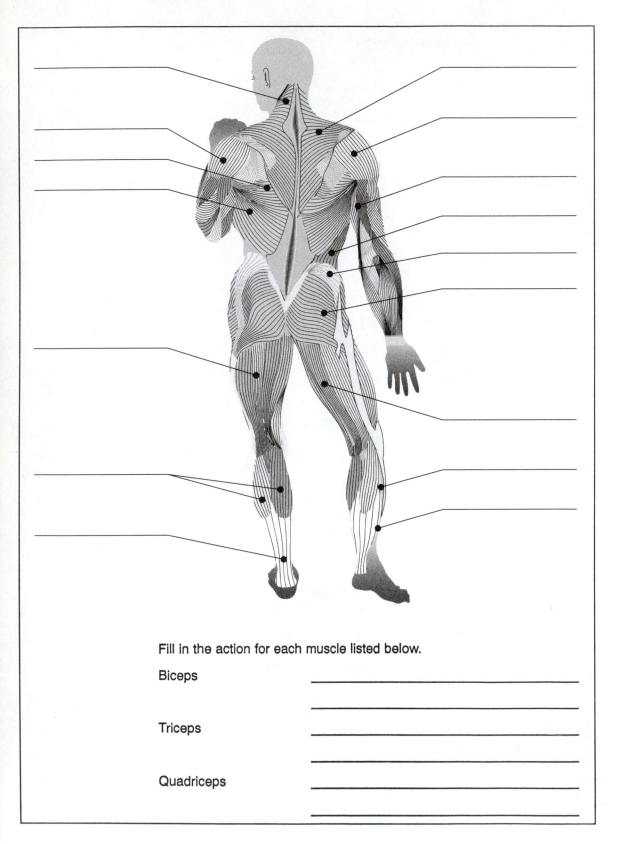

Fill in the action for each muscle listed below.

Biceps _____

_____

Triceps _____

_____

Quadriceps _____

_____

Hamstrings

_____

_____

Pectoralis

_____

_____

Rectus abdominis

_____

_____

Transverse abdominis

_____

_____

Obliques

_____

_____

Hip flexor

_____

_____

Somatotypes or Body Types

Each of us is born with a genetically determined body type. There are three body types (somatotypes): mesomorph, endomorph, and ectomorph. The mesomorph is characterized by a predominance of muscle and bone and is often labeled "very muscular looking." Mesomorphic body types perform best in

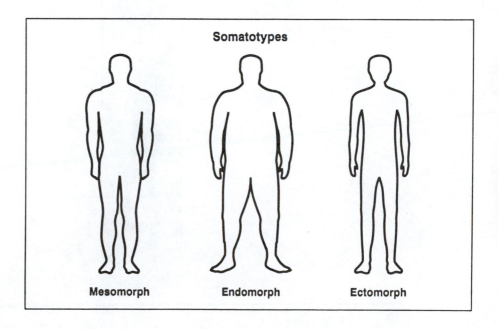

Somatotypes

Mesomorph   Endomorph   Ectomorph

activities requiring strength, speed, and agility. The endomorph is soft and round-looking with an excess of adipose (or fatty) tissue. Endomorphic body types have difficulty performing fast-paced activities. Ectomorphs are very thin and lean. These people do well in endurance activities such as long-distance running and dance/exercise-type aerobics, but may have difficulty in activities requiring strength.

Don't be concerned if you don't fit into one body-type classification—very few people are classified as being strictly one somatotype. Usually a person is a combination of types (such as the mesomorphic endomorph, who appears muscular yet has a rounded look). The significance of this information is being able to recognize that everyone is different. Your goals must be individualized and obtainable, and your objective should be to strive to be the best you can be with the body you inherited.

Body Alignment

While performing all aqua aerobic movements it is important for you to keep your body in proper alignment. Body alignment refers to the position of your body parts in relation to the curvature of your spine. Proper alignment refers to the ideal relationship of all your body parts, with the pelvis resting over the hip joints in a balanced position and the vertebral (spinal) column displaying the normal curves. Maintaining proper alignment will allow your body to perform to its maximum efficiency and reduce the risk of injury.

To test your body alignment, have someone hold a plumb line on your mastoid process (the bone right behind your ear). The line should pass through the center of your shoulder, your hip, the knee area, and the center of your foot.

While participating in your aquatic exercise workout, remember to concen-

Proper body alignment is essential for the safe and efficient performance of all aqua aerobic movements.

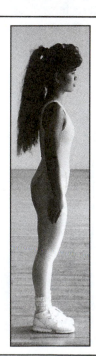

trate on maintaining proper body alignment. A visual image which can help you maintain proper body alignment involves a string attached at one end to the top of your head and at the other end to a helium balloon. Imagine the balloon is pulling you up. This image will help you maintain good posture and proper alignment if you also concentrate on relaxing your hips—don't tuck them under or tilt them back.

Summary

1. You should have some knowledge of basic anatomy for your own interest and so that you can understand your instructor's references to muscles or body areas.
2. Anatomy is defined as the structural makeup of the human body.
3. There are three body types, or somatotypes. They are:
   - mesomorph (muscular).
   - endomorph (round and soft).
   - ectomorph (thin and lean).

4. People are usually a combination of two body types.
5. Body alignment refers to the position of your body parts in relation to the curvature of your spine. Proper alignment refers to the ideal relationship of all your body parts, with the pelvis resting over the hip joints in a balanced position and the vertebral (spinal) column displaying the normal curves.
6. Maintaining proper alignment will allow your body to perform to its maximum efficiency and reduce the risk of injury.

CHAPTER 4

Nutrition and Weight Control

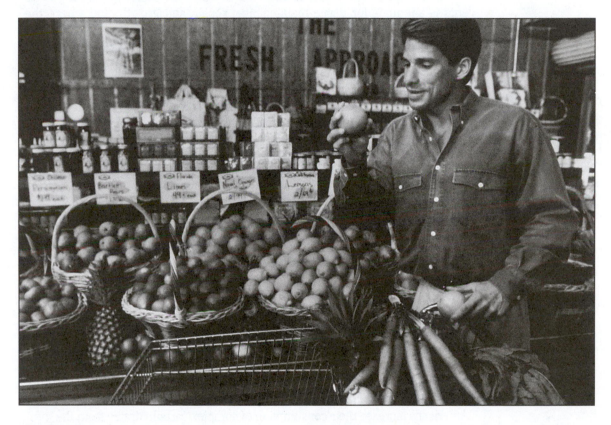

Outline

Basic Nutrition Guidelines

Your body requires a foundation of good nutrition to keep it functioning at its best. Proper nutrition can be accomplished through good judgment in consuming the right amount of carbohydrates, fiber, proteins, fats, water, and vitamins and minerals. Good nutrition is important not only in keeping you healthy, strong, and able to resist disease, but also in controlling your weight.

An optimal diet may be defined as one in which the supply of required nutrients is adequate for tissue maintenance, repair, and growth, and where the nutrient supply comes from a balance of the four food groups. The four food groups are dairy products, protein, vegetables and fruits, and cereal and grains.*

Stick to Variety

Hundreds of gimmicky diet plans come and go, but researchers have found that eating a variety of foods is the most nutritious means of achieving overall health and longevity. A diet deficient in nutrients increases one's risk of developing certain diseases. This is the best reason to avoid fad diets—some can actually be dangerous.

A nutritious diet includes a wide variety of foods from each of the three caloric groups—carbohydrates, protein, and fat—including sufficient vitamins, minerals, fiber, and water. The American Dietetic Association recommends that your total daily calories be 30 percent fat, 15 percent protein, and 55 percent complex carbohydrates.

Carbohydrates

Carbohydrates are the primary energy source of the body. There are two kinds of carbohydrates: simple and complex. Carbohydrates include starch, vegetables, fruit, and all forms of sugar. Important sources of carbohydrates include milk, breads, cereals, pasta, legumes, fruit, and vegetables. The American Dietetic Association and the National Institute of Health recommend that Americans increase their consumption of complex carbohydrates from the meager 25 percent that they've been eating to a level of 55 percent or higher. Carbohydrates provide only four calories per gram and are not as fattening as many people once believed. Carbohydrates are the exclusive fuel for brain function and are stored in the muscles as glycogen, which is used for short-term exercise. Carbohydrates are also "protein sparing," which means that when you consume adequate amounts of carbohydrates, your body is free to use dietary protein for tissue building and repair. Carbohydrate sources are rich in nutrients, such as B vitamins and iron, as well as fiber.

Simple carbohydrates are simple sugars, such as glucose and sucrose, that consist of one or two molecules. They are nutrient-poor and for the most part contribute empty calories. The average American consumes far too much of simple carbohydrates—almost 124 pounds of sugar per year, much of it hidden in processed foods.

*McArdle, Katch, Katch, *Exercise Physiology* (Philadelphia: Lea & Febiger), pp. 9-10, 405-418.

Complex carbohydrates serve as a long-acting fuel for the body. They consist of a long chain of simple sugars and can be recognized as "starchy" rather than sweet. When carbohydrates are broken down in the body to be used for fuel, the energy derived is ultimately used to power muscular contractions and other forms of biological work. Thus, an adequate intake of carbohydrates in the diet is extremely important for an active individual.

Fiber

Fiber is obtained from whole grains, fruits, and vegetables. Fiber includes both the indigestible, crude type found in wheat bran and the water-soluble type found in beans and apples. It is important for promoting satiety, regulating bowel function, lowering cholesterol, regulating glucose absorption, and possibly reducing the risk of certain bowel diseases. In general, Americans need to eat about twice as much fiber as they now do.

Protein

Proteins are made of amino acids, which are the building blocks of tissues, enzymes, hormones, antibodies, and blood cells. Complete proteins (containing all the essential amino acids) are found in cheese, fish, chicken, milk, meat, and eggs. Vegetables and grains contain incomplete proteins, which can be combined with other types of foods to form complete proteins. The recommended daily allowance (RDA) for protein is 1 gram of protein for every 2.2 pounds of body weight (.8 grams for every 1 kilogram). For a 130-pound woman, it is 44 grams; for a 154-pound man, it is 56 grams. The average American diet contains much more protein than necessary. Although protein contributes only 4 calories per gram, many foods that contain protein also contain fat and therefore can increase calorie consumption and contribute to the development of heart disease.

Fats

Fats are an important energy source and body insulator, and are an essential part of cell structure. Some fats are essential for absorption of vitamins A, D, E and K. These vitamins are also an integral part of blood lipids, steroids, cell membranes, and bile. It is important to limit your intake of saturated fats and fats high in cholesterol, since elevated amounts in the bloodstream are associated with heart disease and stroke.

Fats, carbohydrates, and proteins make up the caloric values of all foods. Proteins and carbohydrates each contain 4 calories per gram, but fats are calorie-dense—1 gram of fat contains 9 calories. Therefore, fat-laden meals can add a tremendous amount of calories to your daily intake even though it may appear that you are eating normal quantities of food. For example, a meal consisting of a hamburger, french fries that have been fried in oil, and a saturated-fat milkshake contains four times the calories of a meal consisting of a fresh salad, broiled fish, steamed vegetables, applesauce, and iced tea with sugar. The typical American diet contains too much fat, too many calories, and too few complex carbohydrates.

Low-Fat Dietary Intake Recommendations	
Total Fat	Average of 30 percent or Less of Daily Calorie Intake
Saturated	None
Polyunsaturated	Up to 10 percent
Monounsaturated	Remaining fat calories
Cholesterol	Less than 300 mg. a day

(Source: National Cholesterol Education Program, as reported in the *New York Times*, February 28, 1990, p. A22.)

Checklist: Calories Contained in Food Groups

1. Carbohydrates   4 calories per gram
2. Fat   9 calories per gram
3. Protein   4 calories per gram

Alcohol

Alcohol, though not a food group, is consumed by many people with meals consisting of foods from the above food groups. It contains 7 empty calories per gram.

Water and Hydration

The body generates heat during exercise, part of which must be dissipated through evaporation of perspiration/sweat. Sweat is made up of water, sodium, potassium, and a few other trace elements. For those who participate in aqua aerobics and other aerobic-type exercise classes, it is very important to replace the water. A good rule of thumb is to drink at least eight ounces of water for every hour of aerobic-type activity you participate in. If you're exercising in heat or high humidity, which could be the case in some aqua aerobics classes, you'll need to drink more. Remember that even though you do not feel yourself sweating in aqua aerobics activities, you are. Many exercisers carry plastic sport-drink bottles with them so they can sip water during their workout. Carrying a water bottle would be appropriate in aquatic exercise also; you could place the plastic water bottle near the pool edge and sip from it when necessary. Most dietitians and exercise physiologists agree that plain, cold water is the best beverage to drink to replenish your fluid loss. Sports drinks such as Gatorade, with added electrolytes, are appropriate for strenuous exercise sessions that last over two hours, such as triathlons and marathons. They are not really needed by the average exerciser to replenish lost bodily fluids.

Vitamins and Minerals

If you are in good health and eat balanced meals from all four food groups, it's unlikely that you need to supplement your diet with vitamins and minerals. However, many nutritionists recommend a vitamin/mineral supplement if you tend to skip meals occasionally or do not eat as well as you should. Megadoses of vitamins are not necessary—stay within the recommended daily allowances.

Vitamins and minerals are organic compounds that are not made by the body but are required for growth, maintenance, and repair of cells and tissues. For example, B-complex vitamins help convert carbohydrate particles into energy molecules known as ATP. Vitamins C and E and the mineral iron are also important for exercisers to sustain good health. As your exercise workload increases, adherence to a well-balanced diet grows increasingly important.

Weight Control

Learning how to make proper food choices is the first lesson in weight management. But close on its heels, and gaining more impetus every day, is the importance of an increased level of physical activity as a lifelong tool for weight control.

Many factors influence a person's weight fluctuations. It used to be thought that the simple mathematical formula of caloric intake versus caloric output was the chief determinant of body weight and, hence, weight control. For those individuals close to their ideal weight, the input/output caloric formula still acts as an important energy equation. The theory can be summarized as follows:

1. Ingestion of calories exceeding expenditure of calories equals weight gain.
2. Ingestion of calories less than expenditure of calories equals weight loss.
3. Ingestion of calories matching expenditure of calories keeps weight constant.

Today, however, research has shown that the picture is much more complex. Heredity, set-point theory, brown fat versus yellow fat deposits, altered basal metabolic rate (discussed in the next section), and other factors influence weight control.

Heredity, for example, has definitely gained in importance as a chief indicator of a child's future weight. Studies of identical twins who were raised apart and had very different eating patterns showed that both twins developed similar excessive body fat deposits despite their dissimilar food intake and activity levels.

Set-point theory supports the notion that a body is genetically determined to remain at a certain weight, and that all efforts to increase or decrease that weight are unsuccessful in the long run. Supporters of this theory point to the fact that the metabolism automatically slows down whenever individuals diet, enabling the set-point weight to remain unchanged.

Brown fat versus yellow fat is another theory that supports a genetic predisposition to obesity. People of normal weight supposedly have more brown fat, a type of capillary-dense fat that surrounds and insulates the vital organs and burns deposits of yellow fat as its chief fuel source. Obese individuals, as the theory goes, did not get their fair share of brown fat deposits at birth and, as a result, store yellow fat—the visible type that lies under the skin.

Weight-Loss Diets

The problem with most weight-loss diets is that they concentrate on the wrong end of the energy equation. Simply decreasing caloric intake without increasing caloric expenditure usually does not result in permanent loss of fat. You must expend and/or decrease calories by 500 to 1,000 per day in order to lose one to two pounds per week. A loss of more than two pounds per week is most likely a loss of bodily fluids, not fat. It is interesting to note that 3,500 calories make up one pound of fat.

Rapid weight loss followed by periods of rapid weight gain is an ailment common among affluent Western societies. New evidence shows that this "yo-yo effect" induced by chronic starvation-type dieting followed by a resumption of normal eating habits makes an individual fatter over the years. Your total body-fat percentage climbs with successive dieting, because the body grows alert to the "starvation" period while you're dieting and responds by lowering its metabolic rate. This survival mechanism is similar to the way hibernating animals store fat for the winter.

The goal of the dieter should be to heighten the body's basal metabolic rate (BMR) with consistent exercise, while maintaining sensible, well-balanced nutritional habits. The basal metabolic rate is the rate at which the body burns energy in order to conduct all the maintenance activities of daily life. BMR decreases with age and with reduced body surface area. It is slightly slower in women than in men. Exercise can help speed up the metabolic rate by increasing the amount of lean muscle in the body.

Safe Weight Loss

Safe weight-loss practice requires perseverance and patience, but it also offers a greater probability for success than crash dieting. To lose one pound per week, you should have a net deficit of 3,500 calories. This deficit is best created by expending more energy and limiting your daily caloric intake to 1,200 to 1,500 calories, depending on your current weight, goal weight, caloric expenditure, and gender. Use this formula to determine the number of calories you need to maintain ideal weight: for women, multiply your ideal weight by 16 if you are very active, 15 if you are somewhat active, and 14 if you are not very active. For men, use 17, 16, and 15, respectively.

For example, if you're a woman weighing 130 pounds and you are not very active, you need 130 x 14 = 1,820 calories a day. If you increase your activity by adding one hour of high-energy aqua aerobics each day, you will need 2,020 to 2,120 calories per day to maintain your weight. The caloric expenditure in an aqua aerobics class will vary by the individual and the intensity of the class, but you could very conservatively approximate 200 to 300 calories expended per each one-hour class. However, if you exercise regularly and still consume 1,820 calories daily, the increased energy required for exercising will help you lose weight over time.

Checklist: Calculating Desirable Body Weight

To calculate your desirable body weight:

1. Determine your present weight: _____ lbs.
2. Determine the percentage of body fat you carry, via skinfold or another method. (Discuss with your instructor.) _____ %
3. Select your desired body fat. _____ %
4. Subtract desired body fat from present body fat. _____ %
5. Multiply the percentage of body fat to be lost (answer to Number 4) by your present weight. _____ lbs.
6. Subtract the answer to Number 5 in pounds from your present body weight. This will lead to your desired body weight. _____ lbs.

Summary

1. A well-balanced diet includes a wide variety of foods from each of the three caloric groups—carbohydrates, proteins, and fats—including sufficient vitamins, minerals, fiber, and water.
2. Research indicates that the proportions of each caloric group from which the average American eats today is not particularly healthful. The typical American diet has far too much fat and protein and not enough complex carbohydrates.
3. The American Dietetic Association recommends that your total daily caloric intake consist of 30 percent fat, 15 percent protein, and 55 percent complex carbohydrates.
4. Chronic dieting reduces the amount of lean muscle tissue in the body, which has the net effect of gradually slowing down your body's metabolism (or metabolic engine).
5. Regular exercise adds muscle to the body and increases your fat-burning capacity.
6. A combination of exercise and proper diet can help you maintain or attain your desired body composition.

CHAPTER 5

Motivation

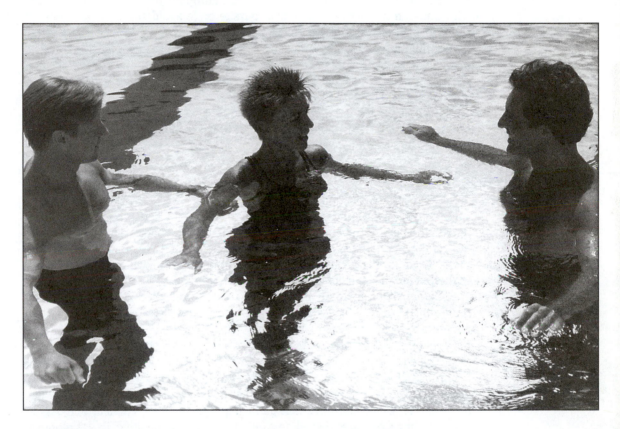

Outline

The desire to become physically fit through aerobic-type exercise often motivates people to begin a regular exercise program. However, this desire to be fit may not be strong enough to sustain them through a long-term commitment to exercise—most people are looking for a "quick fix." Since the results of a regular exercise program don't appear for approximately eight weeks, people often lose their motivation before they see results. In order to stick with a program, exercisers can benefit from a variety of motivating tips and techniques.

Motivation refers to an inner drive that compels you to behave a certain way. You can be motivated either to pursue or to avoid something. Aversion therapy is an example of training the mind and body to be repelled by a negative addiction, such as smoking or alcohol consumption. Incentive therapy involves rewarding yourself with something pleasurable after you've accomplished a certain positive behavior—for instance, buying new clothes after you've trimmed down.

This chapter contains some current thought regarding motivation, from the realm of the sport psychologist. You can use it to help you think about your own motivation as an aquatic exerciser.

Negative Motivation

The motivational technique that may have worked for you at one time will not necessarily motivate you several months down the road. Your attitudes and beliefs about what motivates you are in a constant state of change and adjustment. As you achieve certain short- and long-term goals, what spurred you on in the beginning does not do the same at a later date.

The simplest way to identify your source of motivation is to ascertain and understand your particular needs. Here is an example: Steve is a 24-year-old computer programmer with a sedentary lifestyle and no love of sports. He has been gaining weight steadily and finds himself about 25 pounds overweight. He is surprised to discover that he can't climb the stairs to his apartment without becoming short of breath. The slightest activity seems to wear him out. As he takes a physical inventory, he realizes that he is fast becoming as out of shape as his father, who died from a heart attack at the age of 43. The fear of dying at such a young age scares Steve into signing up at a local health club. He plunges into a six-day-a-week jogging program, develops shin splints from doing too much too fast, and starts to grow discouraged that the weight isn't coming off as fast as he'd like.

The push behind Steve's desire to exercise arose from a negative source: fear of heart disease and early death. Negative motivation isn't without its usefulness—it did get Steve started in the right direction. Many of us experience negative motivation in our everyday lives. For example, you go on a diet because you "can't stand this body anymore," or an eight-year-old finally stops sucking her thumb because she is not going to "let those brats call me a baby anymore."

The negative motivation that drove Steve into jogging also drove him into an overuse syndrome, where he did not approach his fitness regimen with a realistic plan. A painful case of shin splints could keep Steve from jogging for several weeks. This is long enough to set up a cycle of despair, feelings of failure, complete inactivity, and more weight gain. For Steve, overcoming the obstacles to jogging may be more difficult the second time around. He could, however, enter an aqua aerobics class and begin exercising sooner than he could return to jogging. Unfortunately, many people don't realize how valuable an aquatic exercise class can be to them as they are recovering from an overuse injury, such as shin splints.

The problem with negative motivation is that although it may be useful in the beginning, it is often not enough of an impetus to sustain a lifetime commitment. Negative motivation makes you run from something, but not necessarily *to* anything. If the negative event or feeling that originally triggered the action starts to fade from memory or grow distant as time passes, there will not be enough motivation to maintain a strong commitment to fitness.

Positive Motivation

Positive motivation refers to attitudes, beliefs, and traits that spring from a source that enhances your performance, outlook, and confidence about exercise. Although it is more difficult to experience positive motivation in the initial stages of an aerobic-type exercise program (aqua aerobics, swimming, jogging, dance-exercise aerobics, etc.), the nature of positive motivation is more sustaining in the long run.

Here is an example of positive motivation. Karen is a 20-year-old college senior who has devoted all her energy to studying and passing her final examinations. She admits to letting her body "fall apart" by existing on junk food, very little sleep, and a complete lack of exercise. Now that she has to enter the career market, she wants to "clean up her act," as she says, and get in shape for job interviews. As she starts taking aqua aerobics classes three times a week, she finds that they are tougher than she thought they would be. However, she is determined to achieve her goals of a five-pound weight loss in one month, a firmer physique in three months, and more energy.

Karen keeps a weekly log of the time, intensity, and frequency of her participation in aqua aerobics classes, and also records her weight and participation in other exercise-related activities. After three weeks, she is surprised to find that her eating patterns are starting to change. The desire to load up on high-fat fast foods is starting to diminish, as it seems pointless to her to work so hard in exercise class and then counteract all her good efforts with one quick fix of a greasy burger, fries, and a milkshake. The aqua aerobics class is becoming a little easier, but she remembers how tough it was in the beginning.

Karen is not alone. Sports psychologists have studied a transference of positive health habits to other lifestyle aspects among first-time exercisers. People who become committed to their exercise programs tend to cut down on smoking, eat a more nutritious diet, and reduce alcohol consumption and substance abuse.

Positive motivation is self-reinforcing behavior that allows you to continue an action because of the rewarding benefits that slowly become evident. The human body was not made to be inactive, but to be used physically. When we exercise regularly, the bones, muscles, heart, lungs, and blood vessels all begin to function better. If we do not stimulate our bodies into physical action, all of its functional capacities start to decline at an accelerated rate, and we begin to grow old before our time. When the benefits of regular exercise, both psychological and physical, begin to kick in—anywhere from three to twelve weeks after starting an exercise program—positive motivation can take the incentive job over from the initial negative motivation. Positive or intrinsic motivation can last a lifetime.

Inner-Directed versus Outer-Directed Motivation

Have you ever known a person who is self-motivated? Self-motivated people and their personality traits are often the subjects of studies on exercise adherence. One personality trait that distinguishes self-motivated people is their ability to dismiss easily the types of excuses other individuals use to avoid exercise—they don't look good that day, the class is too crowded, they don't feel like going alone, etc. Self-motivated people are inner-directed; their goals come from an inner source instead of from others, such as family and friends.

Outer-directed individuals exercise because their boyfriend or girlfriend wants them to get in shape, because their friends joined a club; basically, to please someone else. The chances of staying with an exercise program are less for the outer-directed than for the inner-directed person. Because there is no conscious awareness attached to the exercise, the outer-directed person does not always look forward to its benefits and often drops out of the program before any real gains are made. It is possible for the outer-directed individual to shift to being an inner-directed exerciser—think of a person you know who started exercising to attract someone's attention, but continued with the program regardless of whether the original motivator was still on the scene.

Why You Keep Going

What really keeps you going in an exercise program? What makes you put on your bathing suit for one more class, even on days when you're dragging your heels? Research shows that for many people, the physical benefit of exercise is stimulus enough to keep them going. For others, the psychological benefits outweigh the physical. But for the majority, a sense of well-being and a positive glow following exercise tend to keep them positively addicted to their exercise regimens.

Traditionally, exercise scientists have looked to the "runner's high" as a reason for long-term adherence. The runner's high, reported by millions of jogging and aerobic-type exercise enthusiasts, is a feeling of elation and uplifted spirits that lasts two to six hours after a vigorous exercise session. Physiologically, it stems from the release of a neurochemical transmitter, known as *endorphin*, which affects the body in a way similar to morphine. All sensation of pain or discomfort is masked, and a feeling of expansive self-worth occurs.

Today, some scientists are reporting that a psychological addiction to exercise kicks in with or without the release of endorphins, and that the positive mental attachment to the entire fitness lifestyle is what keeps people coming back for more. In any case, the mental benefits of aerobic-type exercise carry their own motivational message.

Mental Benefits of Aqua Aerobics

Research in the last two decades has led investigators to conclude that there are mental benefits derived from participation in aerobic-type exercise. These include

- Overall improvement in self-esteem.
- Improved ability to cope with stress and tension.
- Less free-floating anxiety.
- Enhanced ability to focus and concentrate on one issue at a time.
- Increased confidence about reaching goals.
- Greater sense of self-acceptance.
- Greater sense of satisfaction.
- Overall improvement in mood.
- Increased ability to relax.

Many of these mental benefits can enhance your physical performance during aqua aerobics. The improvement in focus and concentration is a good example. If you increase the amount of power that you apply to resisting the water, by pushing harder or making larger movements, you can actually intensify the workload of that area to increase strength, muscular endurance, and total caloric expenditure.

Another example of a mental benefit having an impact on performance is the ability to relax. When you are relaxed in an environment, your performance will be enhanced. Your breathing pattern will work for you by allowing you to inhale fully, which will bring oxygen that the working muscles need into the body. Relaxation also promotes the proper rate of exhalation, which will allow carbon dioxide, a byproduct of exercise, to be expelled from the body. Rest, also an important part of physical training, goes hand in hand with relaxation and can lay the groundwork for your progression to the next level of goal achievement.

Setting Goals

Setting goals and working toward their accomplishment is a significant part of all exercise programs, including aqua aerobics. Goal setting also goes hand in hand with motivational techniques. The gratifying sense of achievement that follows when a goal is accomplished scores high marks as a motivational tool. That success can be transferred into all other areas of life that impact your exercise regimen, reinforcing the next wave of goals and efforts.

Goals for an aqua aerobics program might include

- To gain both strength and cardiovascular endurance.
- To develop more power.
- To gain greater flexibility.
- To reduce your percentage of body fat.
- To lower your resting heart rate.
- To sleep more soundly, owing to the right amount of physical fatigue.
- To feel better.
- To look better due to improved muscle tone.

- To relieve stress.
- To improve your overall health.

Following the Goals with Action

Motivation centers around the intensity and extent of your desire to accomplish a goal. The amount of enthusiasm you have in pursuing a goal indicates how much you really want to achieve that goal. Many people say that they want to accomplish a goal, but only by looking at how fervently they pursue it can we accurately measure their desire for a positive outcome. It's not enough to say "I want to get in shape;" what counts most is your demonstration of setting measurable, realistic objectives of small increments that will help you move toward achieving your goal(s). With exercise, the action rather than the expression is what matters—it's what you do that counts, not what you say.

Visualization

The practice of imagery or mental visualization is a technique that has been useful in motivating athletes to improve performance. The technique was pioneered by sports coaches in European nations, and has been successfully employed by sports professionals and enthusiasts everywhere.

During mental visualization, the participant usually keeps his/her eyes closed while envisioning the actual performance of a sport or activity, with perfect execution, and a successful outcome. Greg Louganis, the U.S. Olympic champion diver, uses visualization to rehearse a dive, as does golf pro Jack Nicklaus to rehearse a play. As an aquatic exerciser, you can practice your routine mentally by seeing yourself performing the moves correctly. An advanced imagery technique allows you to move the action internally so that instead of closing your eyes and watching yourself do something, try to imagine others watching you flawlessly execute a perfect, high-energy 60-minute class.

The technique of visualization works as a motivational tool because it helps you embrace the concept of yourself as a competent aqua aerobics participant. Once you think of yourself as successful at something, you begin to adopt new attitudes and beliefs about yourself. This is part of the new "you." You can do this easily, with total enjoyment, and have the ability to derive lifelong benefits from exercising regularly in aqua aerobics workouts. Your motivation increases in proportion to your successful achievement of the task.

Additional Motivation Tips

Researchers have found that people who exercise at the same time every day are more likely to stick with an exercise program than people who vary their times. When your exercise facility is convenient to your home or work, you will be more likely to maintain a regular exercise schedule. Another successful motivational technique is to find an exercise buddy. If the social context of exercise is friendly and inviting, the positive feelings are reinforcing. Finally, using a progress log and recognizing your achievement are highly motivational.

Checklist: What Motivates Your Behavior?

To help you assess your motivation and behavior, answer the following questions honestly.

1. Is your motivation to exercise positive or negative?

   _____

   If it is negative, how can you change it to positive motivation?

   _____

2. Are you self-motivated and inner-directed, or outer-directed?

   _____

   If you are outer-directed, how can you change your motivation to become inner-directed?

   _____

3. List three mental benefits you have experienced from exercising.

   _____

   _____

   _____

4. List two goals you have set for yourself that you would like to achieve from participating in an aqua aerobics program.

   _____

   _____

   List two small incremental actions or measurable objectives that you can accomplish in working toward each of the goals listed above.

   _____

   _____

   _____

   _____

5. How can you best use the practice of visualization to help you in your aqua aerobics exercise program?

   _____

   _____

   _____

Summary

1. Try to identify a particular need you have for exercise. Look for something that can be solved or improved through regular exercise.
2. Beginning exercisers can be driven to launch a program because of negative motivation. Although useful, this is often not enough to lead them to a long-term commitment.
3. Positive motivation arises from the self-reinforcing benefits of exercise, both physical and psychological.
4. The inner-directed exerciser is someone who is self-motivated and overcomes the common barriers to working out.
5. Outer-directed individuals may exercise because of someone else (or something else) in the early days of their exercise program, but can then switch their source of motivation to become inner-directed.
6. The psychological benefits of exercise coupled with the release of endorphins create a strong motivational force.
7. Setting and achieving goals for exercise can trigger feelings of success and self-worth throughout your life.
8. Visualization is a method of mentally rehearsing an ideal performance.

CHAPTER 6

Aqua Physics

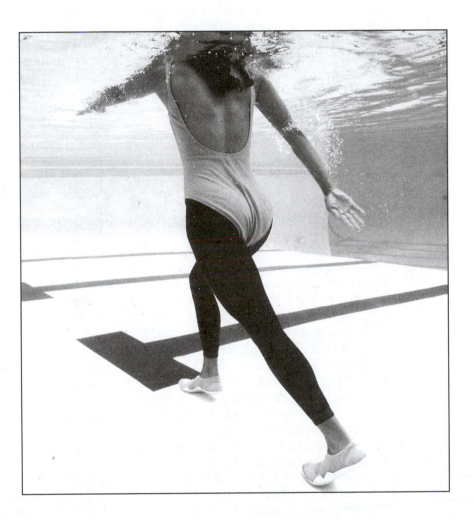

Outline

Working out in the aquatic exercise environment requires some knowledge of what is commonly called *aqua physics*. This chapter will provide you with basic information in this area.

Newton's Laws of Motion

Aqua physics is the application of the physical properties of water, including Sir Isaac Newton's laws of motion (defined in the 17th century), to aquatic exercise. Newton's first law of motion states that an object remains either stationary or moves at a constant velocity unless acted upon by a force. Pressure of the hand/arm and foot/leg surfaces causes body motion or changes the speed and direction of motion. Resistance of the body to any change of motion is known as *inertia*. An aqua aerobics application of the first law of motion would be that a stationary aquatic exerciser must provide a force in order to overcome stationary inertia and move through the water. Once in motion, the exerciser needs to continue the movement patterns in order to maintain the motion. A slowing down of the movement and a loss of the forward momentum, called an *inertia lag*, requires extra energy to put the body in motion again.

The second law defined by Newton, the law of acceleration, explains the relationship between the force that is applied by an exerciser and the changes in motion that result. This law states that the acceleration of an object depends upon its mass and the applied force. The formula for this law is: acceleration equals force divided by mass. Applying this law to movement in aquatic exercise, a strong person jumping forward through the water will cover more distance than a weaker person with the same body weight because the individual with the stronger muscles will be able to apply more force and thus move his/her body further and faster (velocity) than the weaker individual. Exercisers who are heavy have more mass to push through the water, and need more strength (force) in order to cover the same distance in the same amount of time as a lighter exerciser with less mass. The law of acceleration can be applied to your workout and be used to increase or decrease the intensity. Applications include pushing off the bottom of the pool with great force to cause your body to spring up higher and faster, pulling or sweeping your arms through the water with great force in order to travel through the water farther and faster, and taking larger steps in the same amount of time to add greater force and intensity to your workout.

Newton's third law of motion governs movement through the water: for every action there is an equal and opposite reaction. To walk or run forward in the shallow water you need to push back and down against the pool floor with alternate feet. The pool floor produces the reaction force, which acts in opposition to your own force in order to create forward movement. The harder you push back, the more forcefully you will move forward through the water. To move through deep water you must use large pedaling-type movements, simulating an astronaut walking through space. The forward momentum is produced by extending the ankles to press the foot surfaces alternately downward and backward through the water. Use of the arms and hands in a dog paddle or sculling-type action also provides support and forward propulsion for the body. Again, the harder you pedal and paddle, the more forcefully you will move through deep water.

Body Surfaces, Water Resistance, and Energy Expenditures

The broader the surface of the body part that you use to push or press through the water, the greater the water resistance to that body part. Conversely, when the body surface is narrowed during aquatic exercise, the resistance to movement of that body part will decrease. For example, pressing through the water with scooped hands will offer greater resistance than slicing through the water with the little fingers or thumbs leading. Therefore, using broad surfaces of your body to press and pull through the water will increase water resistance to the body and increase the energy expended in movement. In order to conserve your energy and decrease the water resistance, use narrow body surfaces to move through the water.

Eddy Resistance

As the body moves through the water, a certain amount of drag or *eddy resistance* occurs. Eddy resistance is caused by clothing worn over bathing suits, resistance equipment, and the shape of the body part moving through the water. A straight limb slicing laterally through the water will create less eddy resistance than a bent one.

Principle of Leverage

The human body is composed of a system of levers that function to produce force. Many of the movable joints in the body act as what are classified as third-class levers. The joint is the fulcrum of the lever, and the effort is applied at the point where the working muscle is attached to the moving bone.

The resistance arm of the lever is the distance from the fulcrum or joint to the place where the resistance is felt. In aquatic exercise, the water itself is the resistance. Water offers 12 times the resistance of air. When you push or pull the water, you are moving a resistance. When using levers, the workload can be increased in two ways:

1. By lengthening the resistance arm.
2. By increasing the resistance.

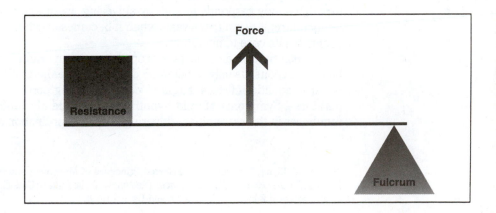

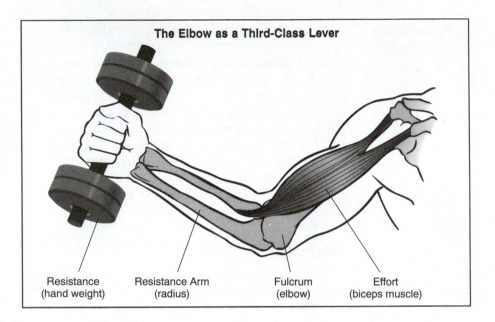

The Elbow as a Third-Class Lever

| Resistance | Resistance Arm | Fulcrum | Effort |
| (hand weight) | (radius) | (elbow) | (biceps muscle) |

Using the principle of leverage in your aquatic workout, you can increase intensity by lengthening the resistance arm and moving fully extended limbs through the water. To reduce the intensity, shorten the resistance arm by bending the knee or elbow.

Absorption of Force During Movement

In all forms of movement your body must absorb the force applied by using a giving action. In aquatic exercise, the force of the body is absorbed by the giving action of the hip, knee, and ankle joints when you contact the pool bottom with one or both of your feet. The giving action of the joints helps to dissipate the downward force of the body and, in conjunction with the cushioning environment of the water, will protect you from injury when landing.*

Thermoregulation

Thermoregulation is the body's attempt to maintain a constant body temperature. The body responds to cold by shivering, in an attempt to warm its core temperature; it perspires/sweats when it becomes overheated, in an attempt to cool down its core temperature.

Hypothermia is defined as a drop in core temperature sufficient to affect bodily functions, usually to below 95 degrees Fahrenheit. Mild hypothermia can occur in aquatics classes taught in cool swimming pools and/or cold air temperatures. Symptoms of mild hypothermia include discomfort from the cold, numbness in the extremities, shivering, loss of coordination and concentration,

*Joanna Midtlyng, "Application of Selected Principles of Movement and Aquatic Skills to Water Exercise," *Water Exercise Teacher Syllabus* (Reston, Virginia: Aquatic Council, American Alliance for Health, Physical Education, Recreation and Dance, 1989).

and slurred speech. Aquatic exercisers need to be aware of these symptoms in order to protect themselves from hypothermia. Treatment for mild hypothermia is to go into a hot bath, shower, or jacuzzi. Afterward, remove your wet clothes, dry off, put on warm clothes, and cover up with a blanket. Rest until your body temperature feels normal again. Note that severe hypothermia can be critical, and emergency medical personnel should be summoned to aid the victim immediately.

Bodily Heat Loss

The body loses heat in four ways:

1. *Convection* occurs when the body comes in contact with air or water that has a lower temperature than the body. When the air/water touches the body, the air/water is warmed and then carried away by a streaming movement.

2. *Conduction* is the transfer of heat energy away from the body by substances with which it is in direct contact. Conduction can occur in any medium. Water's conductivity is 240 times greater than that of air, and therefore water is an excellent heat conductor.

3. *Evaporation* is body heat lost through the evaporation of moisture on the skin (perspiration, splashed-on water) as the air flows over it.

4. *Radiation* is the absorption of heat energy to and from solid objects. An example is the body's increasing in temperature from the sun.

Be sure that your movements throughout your entire aquatic exercise workout are vigorous enough to keep your body in a thermal comfort zone. If you begin to feel cold, increase the speed, size, and force of your movements to maintain a higher workload, which will produce more body heat. Try to keep moving throughout the class. If you are working out in an outdoor pool, try to stay in a sunny area. If you are indoors, keep external doors and windows closed to maintain the ambient temperature.

If you enter the pool fatigued, hungry, dehydrated, having just smoked, or having just had a drink containing caffeine, you stand a greater chance of feeling cool in the water than if you were fully rested, not hungry, or not dehydrated. Protect yourself so you can obtain the maximum benefits from each workout.

Summary

1. Aqua physics is the application of the physical properties of water, including Sir Isaac Newton's laws of motion, to aquatic exercise.
2. Newton's laws of motion have major applications to aqua aerobics. The first law of motion states that an object remains either stationary or moving unless acted upon by a force. The second law, the law of acceleration, states that the acceleration of an object depends upon its mass and the applied force; mathematically, this is described as acceleration equals force divided by mass. The third law of motion states that to every action there is an equal and opposite reaction; for example, to walk or run for-

ward in the shallow water, you need alternately to push back and down against the pool floor with your feet.

3. The broader the surface of the body part that you use to push or press through the water, the greater the water resistance will be to that body part.

4. To increase the water resistance and therefore increase the energy expended in movements, use broad surfaces of your body to press and pull through the water.

5. To conserve your energy, decrease the water resistance by using narrow body surfaces to move through the water.

6. As the body moves through the water, a certain amount of drag or eddy resistance occurs.

7. The human body is composed of a system of levers that functions to produce force. Many of the movable joints in the body act as third-class levers.

8. Using leverage, an aqua aerobics workload can be increased in two ways: by lengthening the resistance arm, and by increasing the resistance. To increase the intensity of your aquatic exercise movements, lengthen the resistance arm by moving fully extended limbs through the water. If a reduced intensity is desired, shorten the resistance arm by bending the knee or elbow.

9. In aquatic exercise, the body's force when landing on the pool bottom is absorbed by the giving action of the hip, knee, and ankle joints.

10. Thermoregulation is the body's attempt to maintain a constant body temperature.

11. Hypothermia is a drop in core temperature sufficient to affect body functions, usually below 95 degrees Fahrenheit.

12. Symptoms of mild hypothermia include discomfort from the cold, numbness in the extremities, shivering, loss of coordination, loss of concentration, and slurred speech. Aquatic exercisers need to be aware of these symptoms and protect themselves from hypothermia. Treatment for mild hypothermia includes getting the individual into a hot bath, shower, or jacuzzi.

13. The body loses heat in four ways: convection, conduction, evaporation, and radiation.

CHAPTER 7

The Heart of Class—
Aqua Aerobics Movements

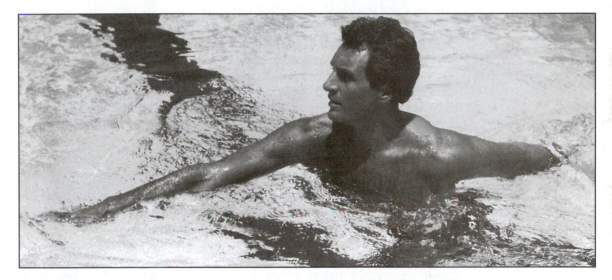

Outline

The movements and activities used in an aqua aerobics class are intended to warm up your body for more strenuous work, give you an aerobic workout, and improve your strength, flexibility, and endurance.

Warm-Up Activities

Most aquatic exercise instructors begin a class with warm-up activities and gentle stretches in the pool. Some instructors have their students begin warm-up exercises and stretches on the deck prior to entering the pool. This land warm-up might consist of walking in place or around the pool deck, and progress to jogging in place. Then the instructor will lead some gentle stretches. Exercise physiologists have demonstrated that flexibility increases only if the muscles are warm. Therefore, any stretching executed with cold muscles will not promote flexibility and could even cause muscle strains. Once you have observed the class you are considering taking or have attended the first class, you will discover which warm-up style the instructor prefers.

Your Pre-Class Warm-Up

It is important to warm up before you exercise, to prepare your muscles and joints for a strenuous exercise session. During the warm-up, you need to raise your heart rate gradually and warm up the major muscle groups. You need to allow yourself about nine to fifteen minutes for a good overall body warm-up. If you are taking an aqua aerobics or aquatic exercise class, your instructor should lead you through an appropriate warm-up routine. The first three to five minutes of a warm-up led by the instructor in the pool is called a *thermal warm-up*. Its main purpose is to warm up the major muscles, which will allow the body to deliver extra oxygen to the muscle tissues and thus prepare them for a vigorous workout. However, some people like to warm their bodies up gradually before entering the pool or taking a class. A simple way to do this is to walk around the pool deck or exercise facility, and gradually increase the pace.

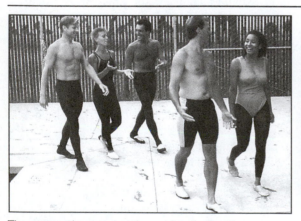

The warm-up in some aquatic exercise classes begins with a walk around the deck.

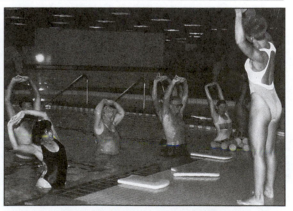

A thermal warm-up raises the heart rate gradually and warms up the major muscle groups to prepare the body for a vigorous workout.

Then you can ease yourself into the pool and begin walking through the shallow water, gradually walking faster and faster. A large muscle (or gross motor) warm-up is necessary to prevent muscle tears and strains. Once your body has warmed up a bit, stretching slowly and gently before class may make you feel ready to begin the class with more vigor. After walking around the deck (and perhaps in the shallow water), doing some of the following would comprise a good pre-class stretching session.

Caution

Be sure to use correct technique when walking and jogging through the water—use the same heel–toe foot action when walking or running through the water as you would on land. Some people have a tendency to jog through the water or in place on their toes, which could lead to pain and injury due to the shortening of the gastrocnemius and soleus muscles that occurs when you move only on your toes.

Stretches and Isolations

Overhead Stretch

Stand with your legs shoulder-width apart and your knees slightly bent. Alternately stretch one arm and then the other overhead toward the sky and hold it for eight counts. Repeat two times.

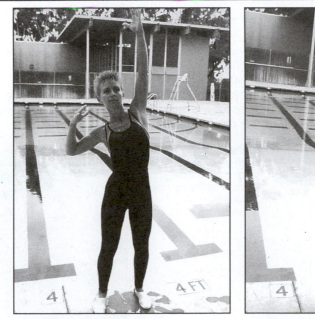
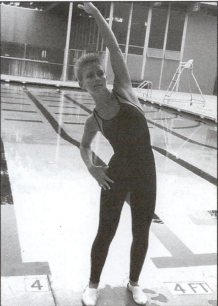

Overhead stretch   Overhead side stretch

Overhead Side Stretch

Stand with your legs shoulder-width apart, your knees slightly bent, and your toes turned out. Alternately stretch the right arm and then the left overhead on a diagonal while the opposite hand rests on the thigh. You should feel the stretch down the entire side of your body. Hold the stretched position for eight counts, and then perform the same movement on the other side. Repeat two times.

Head Isolation

Tilt your head up and down. Tilt your head right and left (ear approaches shoulder on each tilt). Turn your head to the right and then the left. Repeat the set four to eight times.

Head isolation

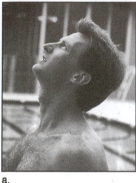 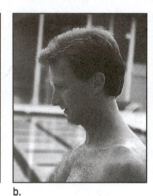 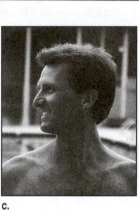 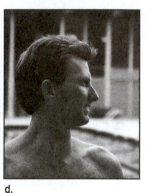

a.   b.   c.   d.

Caution

All head and neck exercises should be performed smoothly and in a relaxed manner. If you allow your neck to arch or roll back, you could put unnecessary tension on the cervical vertebrae. Be sure to keep your shoulders relaxed, and do not shrug them up toward your ears during the movements.

Do not let your neck arch or roll back, thus putting unnecessary tension on the cervical vertebrae.

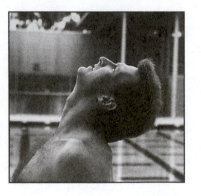

Shoulder Circles

In a slow, smooth manner, circle your shoulders forward, up, back, and around eight times. Then reverse the direction of the roll and repeat eight times.

Shoulder circles

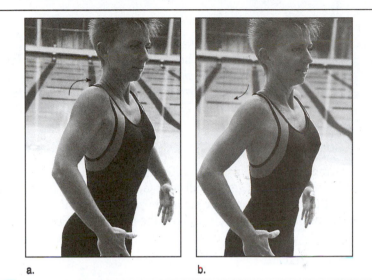

a.   b.

Back Warm-Up Exercise

Bend your knees slightly, and place your hands on your thighs. Begin with a straight back. Contract your abdominal muscles, which will cause your back to round like a cat's. Allow your head to drop naturally, following the action of the spine. Then extend your back and return to the beginning position. Repeat this movement four to eight times.

Back warm-up

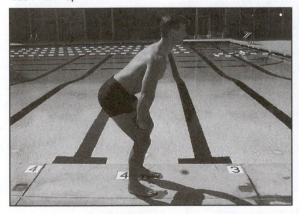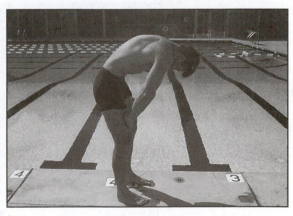

a.   b.

Caution

Keep your movements slow, smooth, and sustained. Jerking movements should be avoided.

Triceps Stretch

Begin with your arms overhead. Bend the elbow of your left arm, pointing the left palm down toward the back of the neck, and hold the left elbow with your right hand. Gently push down the left elbow, which will stretch the triceps muscles. Hold this position for 10 seconds. Perform on the other side. Repeat.

Quadriceps Stretch

Stand up with good posture. Keeping your supporting leg slightly bent, grasp the other leg and gently pull your foot toward your buttocks. Proceed carefully, as this exercise can place stress on your knee joint. Keep your stomach sucked in toward your spine throughout the movement. Perform with the other leg.

Calf Stretches

Perform either or both of the following calf exercises.

- Perform a standing lunge by stepping forward with one foot so that your feet are approximately one to two feet apart. The front leg is bent, and the back leg is straight with the toes facing forward. The heel on the front, lunged leg should remain down, and you should also try to keep the rear heel very close to the floor during this stretch. Hold this position for 20 seconds. Perform on the other leg, and repeat the set.
- Stand facing a wall, approximately two feet away from it. Keep your body in a straight line and lunge forward with one foot, placing your hands on the wall about shoulder level. In the lunge position, your forward leg is bent, and your back leg is straight. You should feel a stretch in the calf of

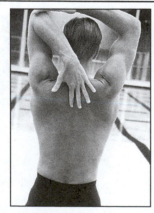
Triceps stretch

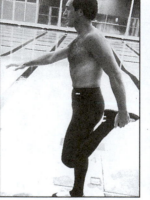
Quadriceps stretch

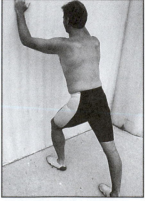
Calf stretch

the straight leg. If you don't, adjust your position by stepping farther away from the wall until you do. Perform on the other leg, and repeat the set.

Groin Stretch

Take a large step to the left, keeping your feet parallel. Bend your left knee and keep your right leg and knee straight. If necessary, place your hands on your upper thighs for support and balance. Hold this stretch for at least ten seconds. This will stretch the right groin area. Repeat on the other side.

Abductor Stretch

Stand on your left leg. While keeping your torso upright, lift your right leg, bent at the knee, up and in across your body. If balance is a problem, you may hold on to the wall (if you are not in the water) or the side of the pool with your right hand for support. Place your left hand on the outside of your right knee and gently press your knee toward your body. This exercise will stretch the abductor muscles on the outside of the right leg. Hold the stretch for 20 seconds. Repeat on the other side.

Ankle Circles

While standing or sitting, circle your ankles slowly and smoothly 10 times in each direction. Repeat.

Ankle Raises

From a standing position in good alignment, raise yourself up onto the balls of your feet (relevé). Hold for four counts, and then lower yourself back to the floor in four counts. Repeat 10 times. Do another set, holding for two counts in each position.

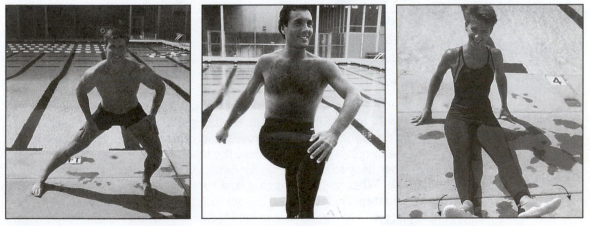

Groin stretch   Abductor stretch   Ankle circles

Caution

When raising up to the balls of the feet, be careful to keep your weight on your big toes so as not to pronate toward the lateral side of the ankle.

Heel Walking

Lift your toes up and walk around in the pool or on the pool deck on your heels. This strengthens your tibialis muscles.

The exercises just described will help prepare you for safe participation in your aquatic exercise class. As mentioned in the opening of this chapter, some instructors will include similar exercises in their class and therefore you may not need to perform them on your own. Others may not, and you may prefer to execute these before the class begins. Since these exercises will help you feel good before you begin your class or get into the water, you may want to execute them in any case.

Heel walking

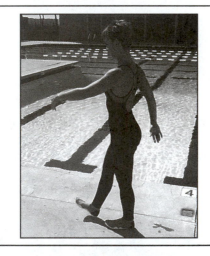

In-Pool Aqua Aerobic Activities

In-Pool Warm-Up Activities

As mentioned earlier, a pre-class warm-up is advisable. For the in-pool warm-up, you should begin with your body submerged in the pool chest-deep. Start by walking through the water and progressively increase your speed. This gradual increase in movement will increase the blood flow to the working muscles and help your body adapt to the demands placed on the circulatory system during exercise. When walking, jogging, and running through the water, be sure to use the natural heel-toe action of your foot that you use on land. When jogging in place or leaping, be sure to land toe-heel with "soft" ankles and knees. The softening or giving action of the feet, ankles, and knees helps safely and efficiently to absorb the force of your landing. Then jog easily in place for one minute, pumping your arms in a natural movement. Increase the tempo to running while still pumping in a coordinated manner as if on land. Jumping, jogging, twisting, hopping, leaping, and lunging activities can be alternated to compose a nine- to fifteen-minute warm-up. The in-pool warm-up is divided as follows:

Thermal warm-up	Three to five minutes.
Pre-stretch	Three to five minutes.
Cardiovascular warm-up	Three to five minutes.

Walking

Take very large walking movements through the water and use your arms to pull yourself through the water. Move your arms in opposition to your legs, as you would when walking on land.

Lunging

Take large lunging steps through the water, moving forward and backward. Use your arms to help pull yourself through the water.

Jogging

Jog in place or through the water while adding the following arm movements:

- Shoulders rolling while jogging.
- Arms pumping while jogging.
- Arms swimming forward through the water, as if executing the front crawl, while jogging.

Walking

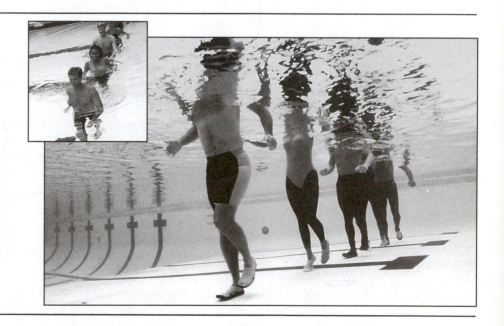

Jogging

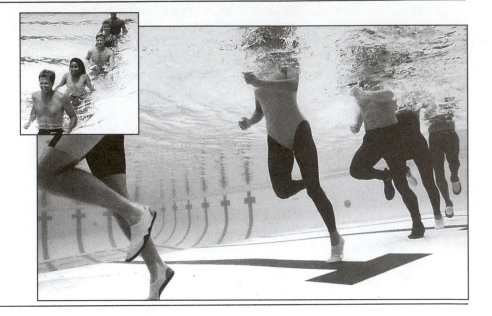

Jogging Backwards

Jog through the water backwards, using arm movements similar to those of the back crawl.

Leaping

- Leap forward from one foot to the other through the water, moving the arms in opposition as if performing the front crawl.
- Leap on a diagonal through the water, with your arms scooping and helping you progress forward.

Caution

When executing jumping movements, be sure to:

1. Land with "soft" ankles and knees to cushion the back and to absorb the force of the landing.
2. Maintain proper body alignment in all movements.
3. Keep the knees in line with the toes.

Jumping

Jump in place with your feet together, keeping your arms to the side. Or, try the following variations:

- Jump in place with your feet together and scull with your arms. To scull, begin with your hands near your thighs. Turn your palms over and push

the water about 1 foot away from your thighs. Then rotate your arms and palms again, and push the water toward your thighs. Keep your arm movements smooth and flowing.
- Jump from side to side, scooping your arms in coordination with the direction in which you are moving.
- Jump in place while punching your arms overhead toward the sky.

Twisting

- Jump and twist your body, with your arms moving at chest level in opposition to the twisting movement.
- Jump and twist with your arms overhead and out of the water.

Jump with arms at sides

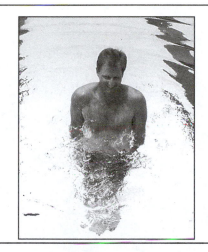

Jump with arm scoops

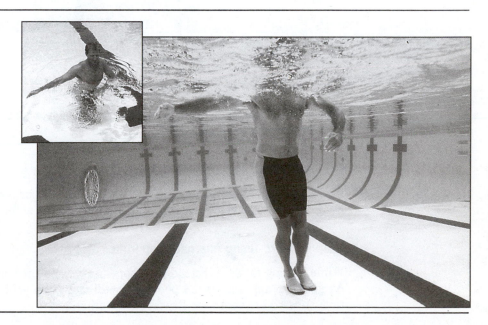

Aerobic Movements

The next section of class lasts approximately 30 minutes and focuses on working your cardiovascular system. It is usually called the *aerobic* section of class. During the aerobic portion of the class, the movements just described for the in-pool warm-up can be performed at a faster pace and in different patterns.

In addition, you can do a combination of the movements that follow.

Running with Arm Scoops

Run in place and alternately scoop arms from side to side through the water.

Run with arm scoops

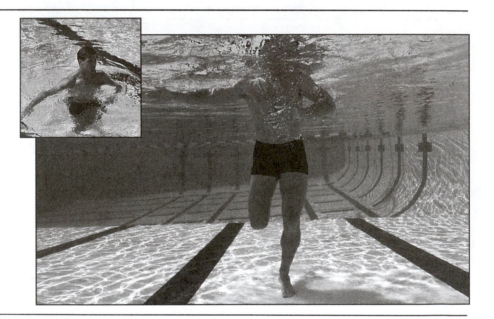

Run Forward and Make Front-Crawl Movements

While running forward through the water, perform front-crawl/dog-paddle-type arm movements with your arms in the water.

Run Backwards and Make Back-Crawl Arm Movements

While running backwards through the water, use the back-crawl arm motion but keep the recovery of the arms close to the surface of the water.

Leap Forward Using Alternate Arm Pulls

While leaping forward, extend your opposite arm on the surface of the water. As your leg approaches the pool floor, pull and push your arm through the water toward the pool floor. Repeat on the other side.

Run backwards with
back-crawl arm
movements

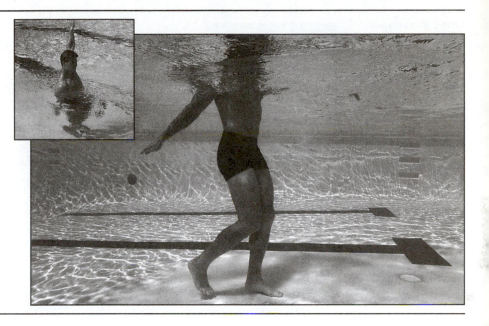

Diagonal Leap Using Double Arm Pulls

Perform the leap forward using simultaneous double arm pulls while traveling on a diagonal path.

Leap Backwards and Scoop with Both Arms

Leap backwards onto one leg. Simultaneously scoop both arms back behind you and finish the arm movement in front of your body. Repeat, leaping onto the other leg. The double arm movement is performed simultaneously on each leap.

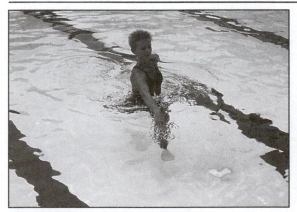

Leap forward with alternate arm pulls

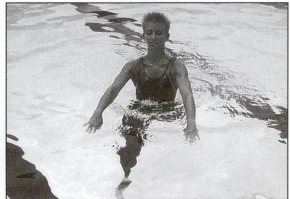

Leap diagonally with double arm pulls

Leap backwards with
arm scoops

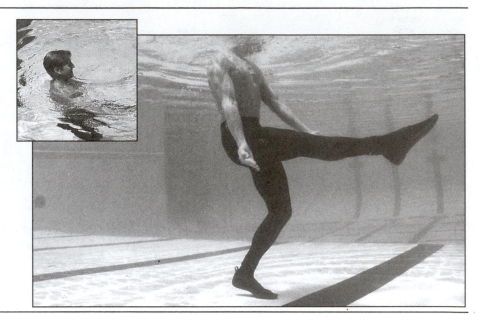

Cat Leap (*Pas de Chat*)

Begin with heels touching and toes turned out on a diagonal. Bend the right leg
so the right toe touches the left knee. Extend the right leg to the side horizon-
tally. Leap to the side onto the right foot. While the right leg is moving through
the water executing the leap, push off with the left foot, bend the left knee so
that the left foot nearly touches the inside of the right knee, and end with the
left foot landing in front of the right foot. Repeat on each side or perform several in a row in each direction.

After you become proficient at this movement, you can push off the ground
and bend both legs simultaneously, the right leg continuing to lift so that the
right toe touches the left knee. This is reversed to begin on the left side.

Cat leap

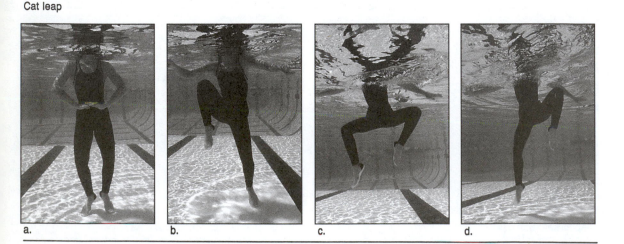

a.   b.   c.   d.

Frog Leap

The frog leap is similar to the cat leap, but it is done in a parallel position. Begin with your weight on your left leg and foot. Lift your right knee bent and move it up and to the side as if you were leaping over a rock and landing to the right side of it. Simultaneously push off the bottom of the pool floor with your left foot and lift the left leg up as high as you can to "get it up over the rock" before it rejoins the right foot on the pool floor. Land with the knees bent deeply. Repeat leaping five times to the right and then reverse, moving to the left. Moving left and right equals one set. Repeat two sets of frog leaps.

Mountain Climber

Begin in a lunge position with one leg in front of the other. Push your body up through the water and change the leg position so that you end in the lunge position with the opposite leg in front. Use your arms in opposition, pushing through the water.

Mountain climber

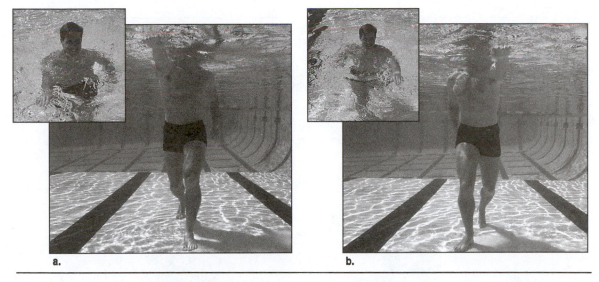

a.   b.

Echappé

Begin with your feet together. Jump to a position in which your feet are just a little wider than shoulder-width apart. Return to the starting position. Repeat in a flowing, continuous manner. This can be done with the feet parallel or turned out, as in ballet.

Pony

Hop to the right onto the right foot, bring the left foot next to the right foot, and quickly step first left, then right. Hop to the left onto the left foot, bring the right foot next to the left, and quickly step right, left. Move your arms in opposition, with one toward the sky and the other toward the feet.

Echappé

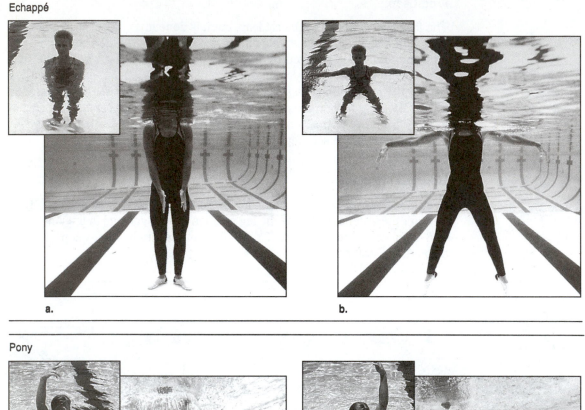

a.   b.

Pony

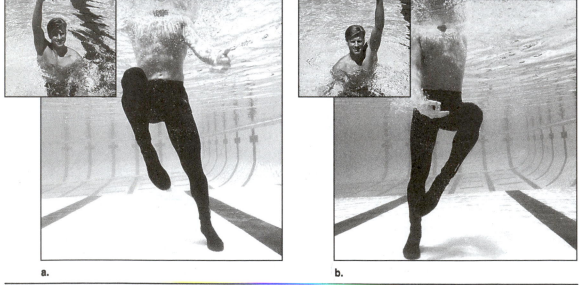

a.   b.

Rocking Horse

Begin with one foot in front of the other. Lift up the leg in front. Rock onto the front foot and then onto the back foot. Repeat several times and then change to perform the rocking action with the opposite leg in front.

Variation: Double Rocking Horse. Rock twice on the front foot and then twice on the back foot. Arms begin bent, with hands up toward the sky and elbows just touching the surface of the water. As the rock goes forward the arms press forward and down through the water. During the rock backwards, turn the palms up toward the sky and pull the hands up through the water to the starting position.

Variation: Kick Up in Front. When your weight is on the back/rear leg, straighten the front leg and kick it up through the water toward the surface. Be sure to execute this variation on both sides of your body.

Caution

Keep your back straight and your abdominal muscles pulled in toward your spine throughout the movement. Just kick as high as your body will allow without any straining.

Rocking horse

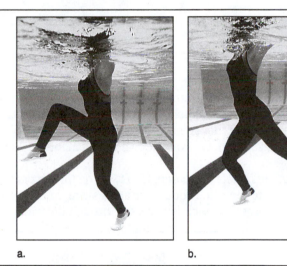

a.   b.

Slides to the Side

Slide to the side and exaggerate the movement when you bring your legs together. You will need to transfer your weight to the leg you initially move to the side and scoop your trailing leg toward the stepping leg. Leave your arms to the sides or simultaneously scoop both arms. As with the cat leap, slides to the side can be repeated on each side. Usually, several slides are performed in each direction.

Leap to the Side

Leap to the side. Cross the trailing leg slightly in front of the leading leg when you land. Use the arm on the same side as the leading leg to scoop and pull you in the line of direction. After several continuous leaps in one direction, change directions.

Slide to the side

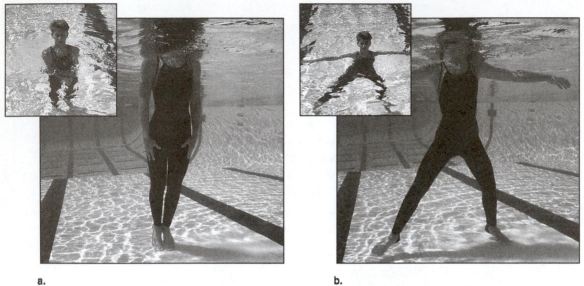

a.   b.

Pendulum

Hop from one leg to the other while the nonsupporting leg swings to the side in a pendulum motion; push the water with the side of the working leg. Push the water down with alternate hand motions as if dribbling a basketball. The arms can also push the water down simultaneously. Repeat in a continuous manner.

Variation: Double Pendulum. Hop twice on the supporting foot before changing support to the other foot. Your arms swing in front to the body and press through the water as each leg presses through the water.

Pendulum

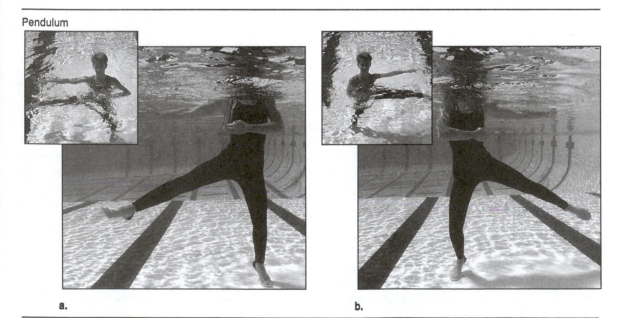

a.   b.

Gallop Forward

Gallop forward, leading with the same leg. Use an arm motion where the arms and hands are pushing the water down toward the thigh as if slapping it. Change the leading leg and gallop forward leading on that leg.

Caution

Participants with ankle, knee, and hip problems should exercise caution in all jumping movements. If it hurts you to perform the movement as the instructor is demonstrating it, reduce the intensity of the activity by jumping lighter or smaller or not at all. If you feel pain, stop doing the movement and consult your physician!

Gallop forward

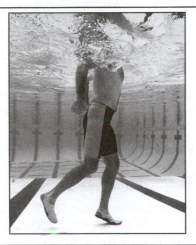

Jump In Place

Jump in place, trying to push your body high out of the water. Use the arms to push down on the water to help move your body up in a bobbing motion.

Jump, Twist with Feet Together

With your feet together, jump and twist your body through the water in one direction and then the other. Move your arms at shoulder height simultaneously through the water in the direction opposite where your lower body is twisting, so that your hips and shoulders are always moving in opposition to one another. Push the water with your hands and forearms. Keep your knees slightly bent throughout the movement.

Jump, Twist with Feet Apart

Perform the jump, twist with feet together movement, except begin by spreading your feet shoulder-width apart. Execute the movement with your knees

Jump, twist with feet together   Jump, twist with feet apart

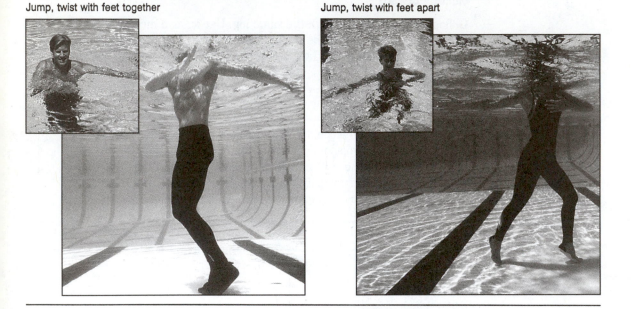

bent a little more than in the jump, twist with feet together exercise. Exaggerate the movement more than in the previous version.

Step, Hop Traveling Forward

Step and hop forward on your right foot while lifting the left leg, bent to the back in a dance attitude position. Then repeat the movement beginning on the left foot. Move your arms in opposition to the leg movement. (As a guide, imagine yourself taking long ice-skating steps while performing this movement.)

Step, Hop, Cross Over to the Side

Step and hop to the right on the right foot while lifting the left leg up to the side, with the knee pointing up toward the surface of the water and the toe pointing down toward the bottom of the pool. Then cross the left foot in front of the right and step on it. Arms move in opposition to leg movements and scoop through the water. Repeat the movement several times moving to the right, then reverse it to begin stepping on the left foot and moving to the left.

Heel–Toe Slide

Extend the right heel forward on a diagonal. Drag the right foot through the water and touch the right toe in front of the left foot. Then, beginning with the right foot, slide two times moving to the right. Repeat on the other side.

Hop, Push Foot

Hop on your right foot with the left knee bent, and simultaneously kick your left foot forward on a diagonal path across the body toward the pool bottom.

Step, hop travelling
forward

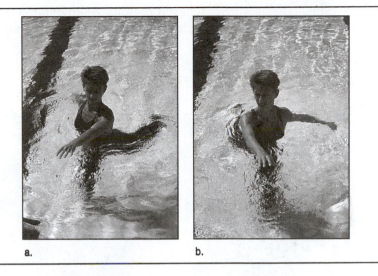

a.   b.

Step, hop, cross over
to the side

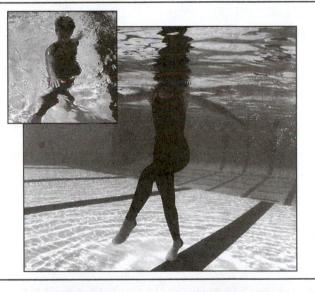

Heel-toe slide

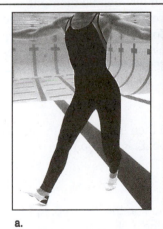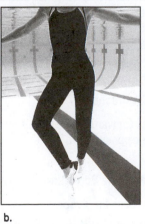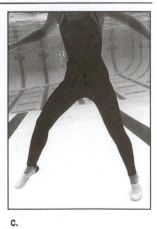

a.   b.   c.

Simultaneously move a flexed right hand through the water on the diagonal toward the extended left leg. Repeat continuously by hopping on the left foot with the right knee bent.

Hop, push foot

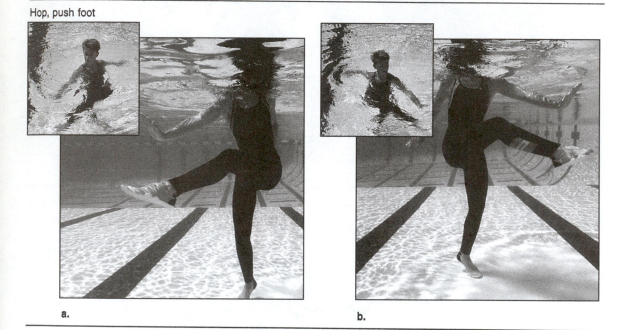

a.   b.

> **Note**
>
> Halfway through your aerobic workout do a pulse check or perceived exertion check.

Grapevine

Step to the right, place the left foot behind the right, and step on it. Then step to the right and place your weight on the right foot. Place the left foot in front of the right and step on it. Continue the pattern and repeat as many times as desired, and then transfer movement to begin with the left foot. Arms can move through the water in opposition to leg movements.

Schottische

Run forward three times and then hop. Repeat the movements beginning with the opposite foot. (R, L, R, hop; L, R, L, hop.)

Grapevine Schottische

Perform the grapevine and hop on the last step: R, L, R, hop. Then repeat the movements on the opposite side: L, R, L, hop.

Grapevine

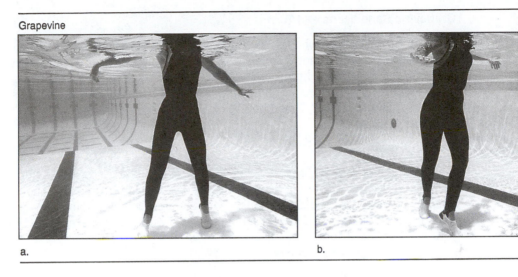

a.

b.

Schottische

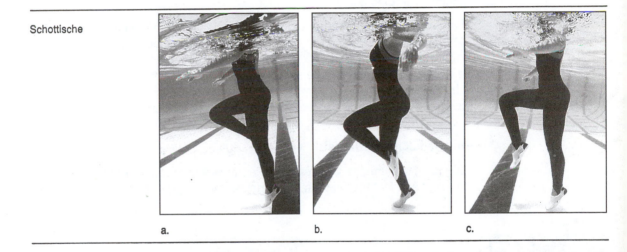

a.

b.

c.

Grapevine schottische

a.

b.

c.

Grapevine Schottische and Turn

Perform the grapevine schottische, but on the hop execute a half turn (180°) to the right so that the movement becomes R, L, R, hop turn, and clap. Then execute the grapevine schottische to the left without a turn. Now, begin the phrase again while you are facing the opposite direction. The movement cues are R, L, R, hop turn; L, R, L, and hop; R, L, R, hop turn; L, R, L, and hop.

Jumping Jacks

Begin with feet together. Jump and then land placing both feet shoulder-width apart. Jump and return your feet to the starting position. Repeat in a continuous motion. The arms move simultaneously with the legs from a position by your thighs to a horizontal position, parallel to the water's surface, and then back by your thighs. The arm movements can vary to make a complete circle, a V, or move in any variety of directions.

Double Jumping Jacks

The timing and the number of jumps are what differ in the performances of a double jumping jack and the jumping jack just described. Begin with your feet together. Jump to the shoulder-width apart position and jump again in that position. Return your feet to the starting position and jump twice in that position. The arms follow right along with the movement in the pattern described for the standard jumping jack but are held during the extra jump.

Inverted Jumping Jacks

The inverted jumping jack places the emphasis of the movement on squeezing the legs and feet together on the jump and pushing yourself off the bottom of

Jumping jack

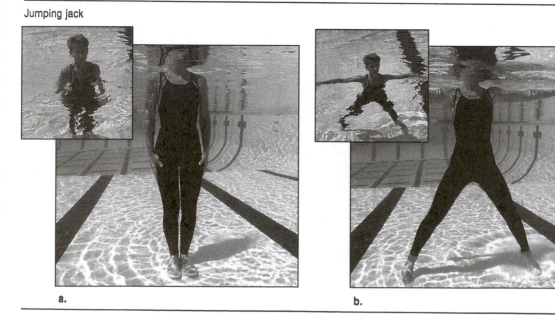

a.   b.

the pool to jump high out of the water. Push your arms toward the pool bottom during the jump to help lift your body out of the water.

Seated Jumping Jacks

The emphasis of this movement is to stay low and squeeze the legs together fast, hard, and with many repetitions. Execute this entire movement with your knees slightly bent, as if you were sitting in a chair. Use your arms to scoop and help you move quickly. When observed from the surface, your head should hardly move up and down at all.

Jump Kick

First jump and kick the right foot forward, then jump and kick the left foot forward. Work arms in opposition by pushing water toward the working foot. Vary the movement by kicking the leg on a diagonal and alternating the direction of the kick. Perform eight jump kicks, alternating sides.

Step, Hop

Step on the left foot and hop on it while simultaneously lifting the right knee, bent, with the foot and toes pointing down. The arms move in opposition, one bent in front of the chest and one straight to the side. Now begin on the right foot and hop and lift the left knee, bent, with the foot and toes pointing down. Repeat many times.

Step, Hop, Jack, Step, Hop

Execute the step, hop movement on the left foot, then do a jumping jack, and then perform the step, hop movement on the right foot. Repeat many times, moving forward through the water.

Inverted jumping jack   Seated jumping jack

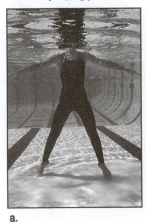 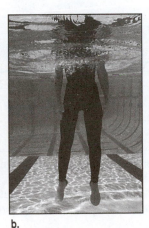 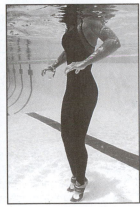

a.   b.   a.   b.

Jump kick   Step, hop

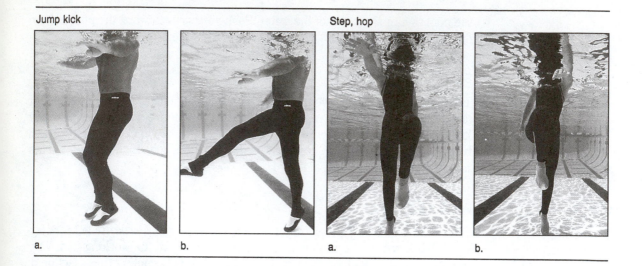

a.   b.   a.   b.

Step, hop, jack, step, hop

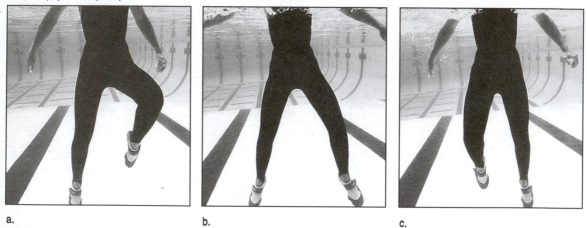

a.   b.   c.

Hop, Touch Elbow to Knee

Hop on the left foot and simultaneously bend the right knee and lift it up toward the chest. When the knee is bent and lifted, touch the left elbow to the right knee, bring the knee down, and jump in place once. Repeat on the other side.

Caution

The object of this movement is to keep the back in an upright position and lift the knee rather than bend forward at the torso. The knee should not be lifted higher than to a 90° angle. Keep your abdominal muscles tight throughout the execution of this movement.

Hop, touch elbow
to knee

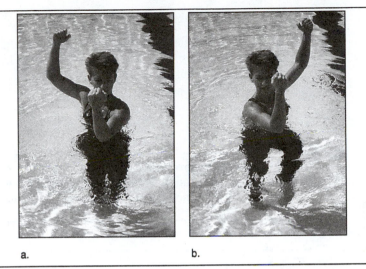

a.   b.

Can–Can Kick

Hop on the left foot and simultaneously bend the right knee and lift it up toward the chest. Hop again on the left foot and kick the right foot out in front to waist height or below, keeping the leg below the surface of the water. Jump in place quickly and immediately begin the movement on the other side by lifting the left knee. Hands can be left on the waist or move in opposition to the legs.

Can–Can Kick and Clap

After you perform the can-can kick movement, clap with both hands under the right leg. Repeat the movement on the other side and clap hands under the left leg.

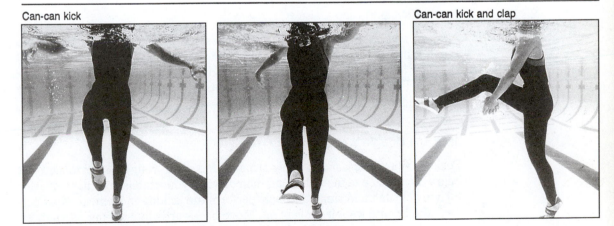

Can-can kick   Can-can kick and clap

a.   b.

Hop, Kick, and Touch Foot

Hop on the left foot and simultaneously kick the right leg to a position parallel to the surface of the water. When the leg is extended in front, reach forward to touch your left hand to your right foot. Repeat on the other side, touching your right hand to your left foot.

Caution

The object of this movement is to keep the back in a relatively upright position and lift the leg rather than bend forward at the torso. If you have difficulty touching your foot, then touch your knee instead.

Hop, kick, and touch foot

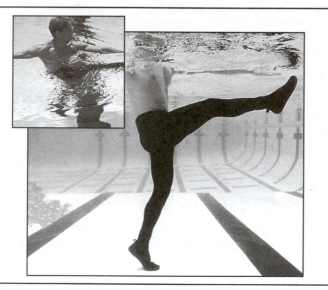

Jump, Kick, and Clap

Jump on both feet. Kick the right leg to a position parallel to the surface of the water. When the leg is extended in front, clap both hands under the leg. Bring the right leg back next to the left and quickly jump on both feet. Immediately kick the left foot in front and repeat the movement on the left side, clapping hands under the left leg.

Jack and Boogie Woogie

Perform a jumping jack and bring arms up and out to your sides, extended just below the surface of the water, and then down to your thighs; execute a quarter turn to your left and simultaneously perform the jacking movement. Next perform the boogie woogie movement. Move backwards by hopping on your left foot and extending your right leg in front, placing your right heel on the floor of the pool. Now hop on the right foot and extend the left leg in front and place

Jump, kick, and clap

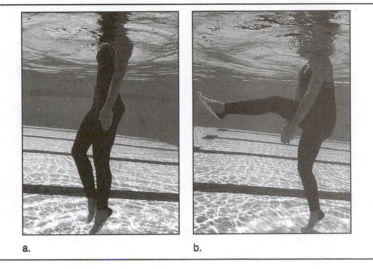

a.

b.

the left foot on the floor of the pool. Repeat the backwards boogie woogie movement two more times (a total of four boogie woogies moving backward). The arms bend at the elbow and push the water down as if bouncing a ball during each boogie woogie movement. The shoulders tilt down as the arms push the water down. Then perform another jumping jack to the left and begin the phrase all over again. You will eventually face all walls of the pool. Repeat the entire phrase several times.

Variation: Begin the movement phrase by turning to the right.

Jack and boogie woogie

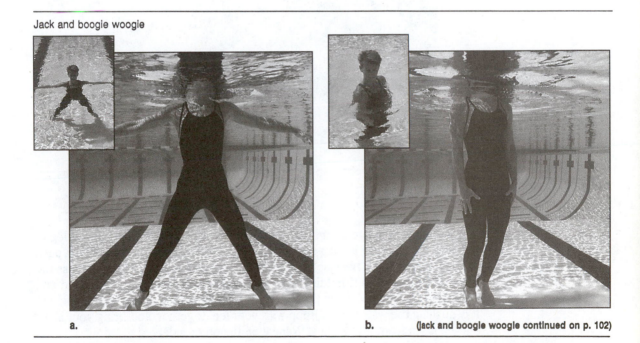

a.

b.   (Jack and boogie woogie continued on p. 102)

Jack and boogie woogie (continued)

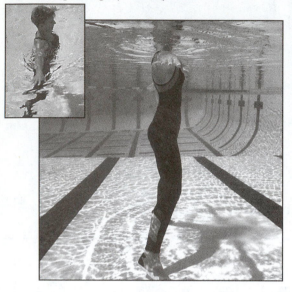

c.

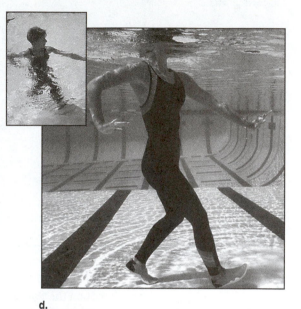

d.

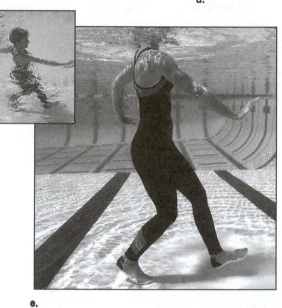

e.

Heel Jack

Hop to the right on your right foot and simultaneously extend your left leg to the side. Keeping the left leg straight, place the left heel on the floor of the pool. While beginning the heel jack, simultaneously pull a bent right arm across the front of the body, as if holding a rubber band in the extended left hand and pulling it across the chest in the right hand. While the left arm is extending out, it is pushing the water back. Jump with your feet together, and bring your arms and hands in front of the chest. Repeat on the other side.

Heel jack

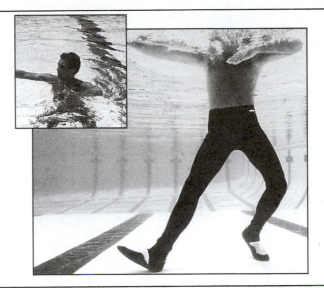

Jack, Kick Back

Perform a jumping jack while extending the arms straight out to the side to a position just below the surface of the water. Execute a quarter turn to the left while beginning a jack facing this new direction. Hop backward on the right foot and kick a left pointed toe through the water on a diagonal to the left, toward the floor of the pool. Flex your right hand and push the water down as if bouncing a ball on the diagonal toward your toe. Perform the same movement on the other side. Repeat the kick movement two more times to perform a total of four backwards hop and kicks. Keep repeating the phrase until you return to the starting position. Repeat the phrase on the other side. This phrase begins with a jack facing forward, a quarter turn to the right to perform the second jack, and a hop and a kick back to begin on the left foot.

Jack, kick back

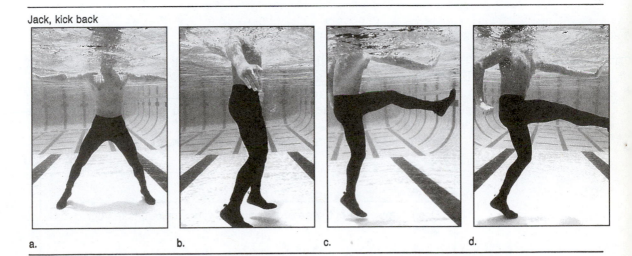

a.   b.   c.   d.

Charleston Bounce Step

Use a very bouncy step throughout this phrase. Step right, kick the left foot forward, step back on the left foot, and touch the right toe to the pool bottom toward the opposite end of the pool. Repeat eight times, and then reverse.

Charleston bounce step

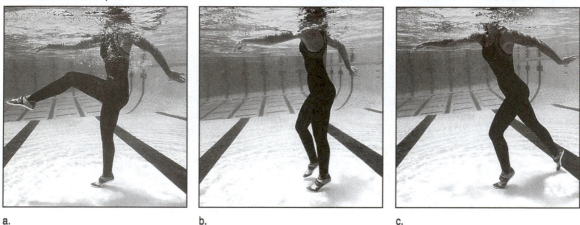

a.   b.   c.

Step, Kick

Take a large walking step through the water and kick a straight leg up through the water toward the surface. When you put the kicked leg down on the floor of the pool, step forward onto it. Repeat on the other side. Arms move in opposition to the legs. Continue this movement until you've traveled the length or width of the pool.

Variation: Reverse the movement, moving backwards through the pool.

Note

Upon completion of the aerobic portion of your workout, take your pulse.

Step, kick

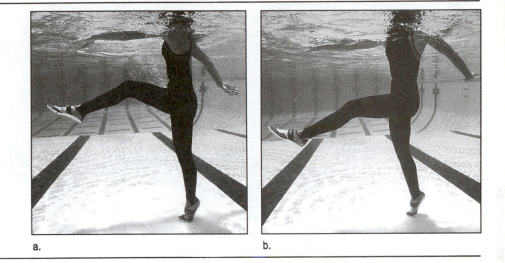

a.   b.

Cool-Down

Following an aerobic workout, it is important to cool down gently using what is called an *aerobic cool-down*.* To do this you can gradually slow down the pace of your aerobic activities and eventually walk around the shallow end of the pool, swinging your arms in opposition while taking long strides. An aerobic cool-down should last approximately five minutes.

Note

Perform a perceived exertion or pulse check at the completion of the cool-down to make sure your heart rate is slowing down.

Upper-Body Strengthening and Toning Work

The following movements are performed to strengthen and tone the isolated upper-body areas. Some of them can be performed simultaneously with aerobic running or jumping activities. Just use your creativity to add interest to your workout.

Breast Stroke—Arms

Begin with your hands touching in front of your chest, elbows up and bent. Stand with your feet shoulder-width apart and slightly bent so that the water is up to your armpit area. Extend your arms in front of your body, and make a half circle with your palms facing down and pulling the water back. When your

*C. Casten and P. Jordan, *Aerobics Today* (St. Paul, MN: West Publishing Company, 1990), pp. 22–23.

Breast stroke—arms

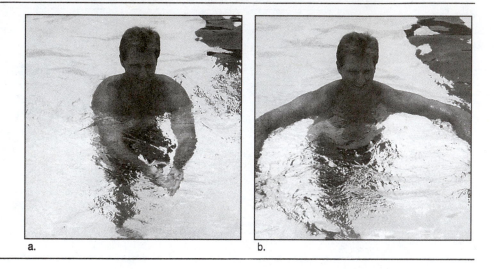

a.   b.

hands have pulled halfway through the half circle, keep the elbows up and pull as if pulling your upper body over a barrel. Return your hands and arms to the starting position and repeat.

This works to strengthen the shoulder area (anterior and medial deltoids), the upper back (trapezius), the chest (pectoralis major and minor), and the front and back of the upper arm (biceps and triceps brachii).

Arm Flies

Stand with your feet shoulder-width apart and your knees slightly bent, in water deep enough to cover your shoulders. Begin with your arms extended to the sides, shoulder height, just below the surface of the water, with your palms facing forward. Bring your arms together in front of your chest and touch your palms together. Rotate your palms so your thumbs point toward the floor of the pool. Reverse the action of the arms by pushing them through the water to the starting position. Rotate the palms so the thumbs are up, to be able to press through the water forward and repeat the movement. Be sure to press through the water with equal force on the forward and backward motions.

This exercise strengthens the chest (pectoralis major and minor), the front and back of the upper arm (biceps and triceps brachii), the shoulder area (anterior, medial, and posterior deltoids), and the upper back (trapezius and rhomboids).

Biceps and Triceps Press

Stand in water that comes up to your armpits. Begin with your legs shoulder-width apart, your knees slightly bent, and your hips relaxed and pointing straight down. Bend your elbows to a 90° angle at about waist level, with the upper arms close to the body and the palms up. Turn your palms over, and press them through the water until the arms are extended behind the body. Rotate the palms to face the pool floor. Press the palms forward and upward

Arm flies

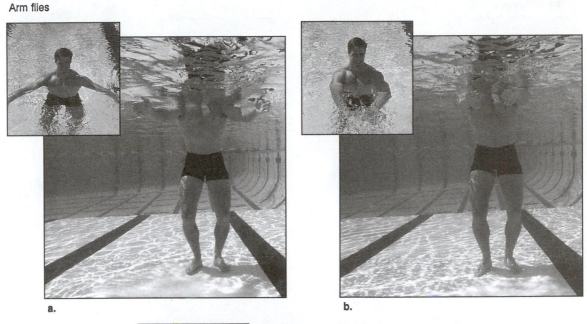

a.   b.

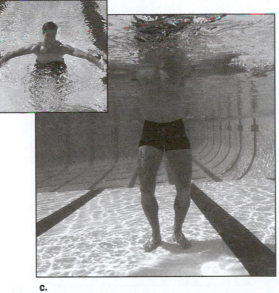

c.

through the water until the elbow is bent and the palms face upward, as in the starting position.

This exercise works to strengthen the front and back of the upper arm (triceps brachii, biceps brachii, and radialis).

Roller

Stand in water that is up to your armpits. Begin with your feet shoulder-width apart, your knees slightly bent, and your pelvis relaxed and slightly tilted under so that the tailbone points down. Bend your elbows and bring your arms to

Biceps and triceps press

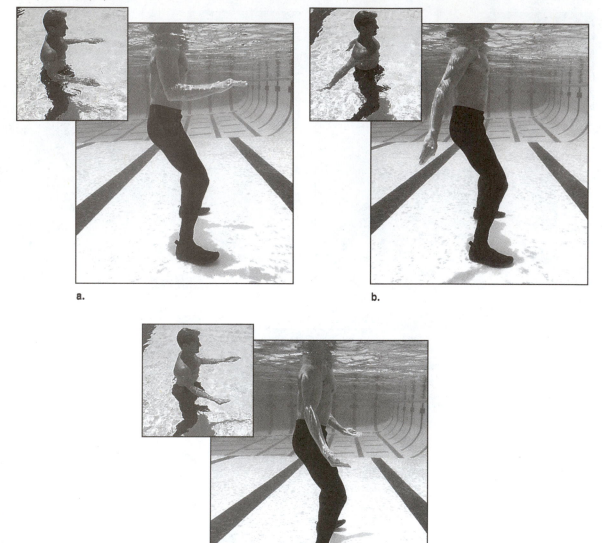

a.

b.

c.

chest height in front of your body with one arm just in front of the other, the hands cupped and facing the body. Rotate your arms in a roller motion, one over the other very quickly and vigorously so that the water really churns. Perform 25 "rollers" in each direction. Repeat.

This exercise strengthens the front and back of the upper arms (biceps brachii, triceps brachii, and brachialis) and the forearm (brachioradialis and the extensor group).

Roller

Roller (side view)

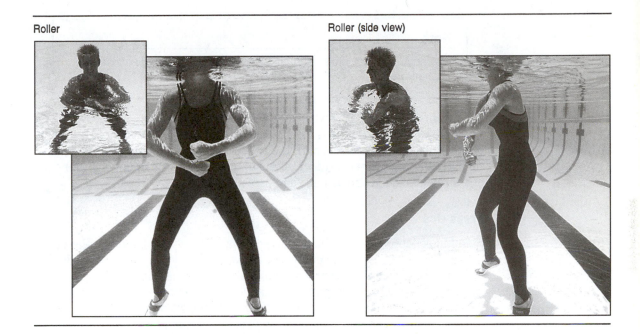

Wall Push-Ups

Stand in the pool facing one of its walls, with the water at the upper-chest level. Extend your arms to place both of your hands on the pool's edge, slightly wider than shoulder-width apart. The feet should be shoulder-width apart, your heels on the pool floor with your toes in line with the knees, and your legs approaching straight but without locking your knees. Keeping your back straight and your feet and knees in a direct line under your shoulders, slowly bend your elbows and lower your body toward the wall. Keep your elbows out to the side. You should feel the weight in your arms and back. Slowly push your body away from the wall to return to the starting position. Be sure to keep your abdominal muscles pulled in to avoid arching your back. Repeat many times and progressively increase your repetitions.

Wall push-up with feet flat

Wall push-up on toes

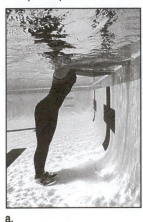
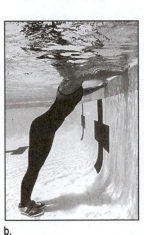
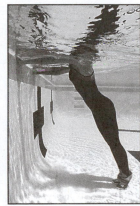
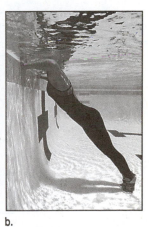

a.   b.   a.   b.

> **Note**
>
> The pace of this exercise can also be slowed down for additional strength training.

Variation: Perform it on your toes with your feet together.

This exercise strengthens the chest (pectoralis major and minor), the front of the shoulder (anterior deltoid), the side of the torso (serratus anterior), and the back of the upper arm (triceps brachii), and also works the Achilles tendon and stretches the gastrocnemius and hamstring muscles.

Press-Ups

Stand in chest-level water, facing the pool wall. Place your hands on the deck near the edge of the pool or on the "gutter wall," with your palms facing down. Your elbows will be bent, your legs straight, and your feet together. Press down on the pool's deck edge or gutter and lift your body out of the water until your elbows are extended. Slowly lower your body to the starting position by bending your elbows and controlling the return. This return movement is the key to the whole exercise—really try to keep the return slow, smooth, and sustained. Be sure to use good body alignment throughout the movement, with your back straight and your head in line with your back. Repeat the movement as many times as you can.

This exercise strengthens the chest (pectoralis major and minor), the upper back (trapezius), the shoulder area (anterior and medial deltoids), and the back of the upper arm (triceps brachii).

> **Caution**
>
> This exercise may not be appropriate for you if you are pregnant, overweight, or are in the "older" crowd and/or have a weak upper body. Consult with your instructor or physician before performing this exercise.

Press-up

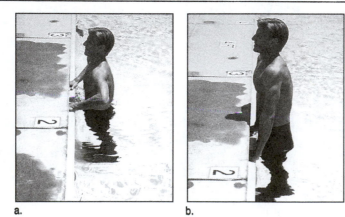

a.   b.

Pectoral Presses

Begin by kneeling down or assuming a low lunge position in the water. Bend your elbows and lift your hands up to face the ceiling. Your hands and arms will make a "U" shape under the surface of the water. You need to be at a level such that just your face is out of the water. Keeping your hands, arms, and elbows moving as a unit, press through the water to bring your arms close together in front of the body, at chest level. Press through the water with the outside of the arms to return to the starting position. This movement simulates the "pec press" Nautilus machine used to strengthen the pectoralis muscles.

Pectoral press

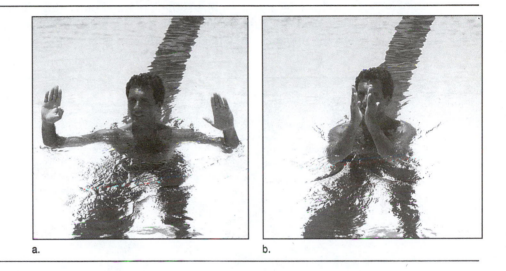

a.   b.

Legwork Exercises

Perform the following legwork exercises in waist-deep water. Stand sideways to the edge/side of the pool and place one hand on the pool's edge. Your other hand may be placed on your waist or out to the side for additional balance.

Side Leg Lifts

Begin with your feet together, body in good alignment, stomach held in, and knees slightly bent. Keeping your toes pointed straight ahead, lift a straight leg to the side. Be sure not to turn (rotate) your hip over or lift it up. You may not be able to lift the leg very high. Pull the leg back down through the water to return it to the starting position. One set consists of 10 to 15 repetitions. Perform one to three sets of this exercise on each leg.

This exercise strengthens the adductor and abductor muscles of the upper thigh.

Side Leg Lift Crossovers

This exercise is similar to side leg lifts, except that you add a crossover in front and in back of your supporting leg on each repetition. Begin with your feet together, body in good alignment, stomach held in, and knees slightly bent. Keeping your toes pointed straight ahead, lift a straight leg to the side. Be sure not to turn your hip over or lift it up. You may not be able to lift the leg very high. Pull the leg through the water towards the supporting leg and cross it in front of the supporting leg until your toe almost touches the side of the pool. Sweep and lift the working leg up and out to the side again and pull it through the water, this time crossing behind the supporting leg. One repetition is the action of lifting the leg and crossing it both in front and in back of the supporting leg. Perform 10 to 15 repetitions on one side before you turn around and begin working the other leg. Executing 10 to 15 repetitions on each side equals one set. Perform one to three sets on each leg.

This exercise strengthens the inner and outer thigh (adductors: magnus, brevis, and longus; gracilis; pectineus; and tensor fascia lata). It also strengthens the upper-hip area (gluteus medius and minimis).

Side leg lift

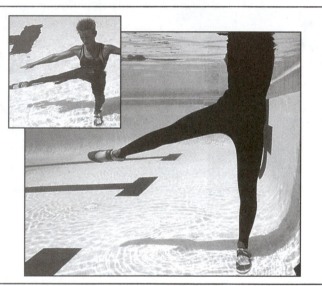

Side leg lift crossover

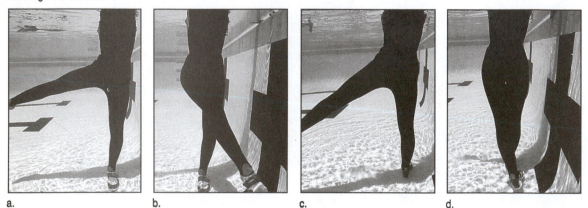

a.   b.   c.   d.

Bent-Knee Side Leg Lifts

Begin with your feet together, body in good alignment, stomach held in, and knees slightly bent. Keeping your toes pointed straight ahead, bend your outside leg (the one farthest from the side of the pool) so that your knees are still near each other but the lower leg is parallel to the bottom of the pool (with toes pointing backward). Now lift your bent leg up toward the surface of the water. As with the side leg lift exercise, be sure to keep your hips pointing forward and do not lift them throughout the exercise. Pull the bent leg back through the water to the starting position. Use equal force in pulling and pushing the leg through the water to gain the maximum benefit from this exercise. Perform one set, or 10 to 15 repetitions, before changing sides. Turn around and perform one set on the other leg. Execute a total of one to four sets per leg.

This exercise strengthens the outer thigh (tensor fascia lata) and the upper hip (gluteus medius and minimis).

Bent-knee side leg lift

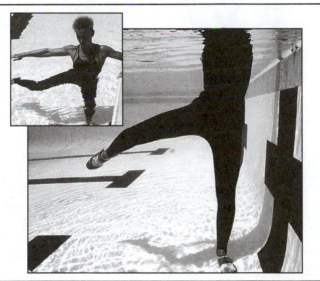

Bent-Knee Side Leg Swings

Begin with your feet together, body in good alignment, stomach held in, and knees slightly bent. Keeping your toes pointed straight ahead, bend your outside leg (the one farthest from the side of the pool) and lift it so that the knee lifts toward the surface of the pool and the toe points toward the floor of the pool. Swing the working foot down through the water, crossing it over the supporting foot, and lift it up to an "attitude" position. Reverse the action by swinging the left foot down and up to return to the starting position.

This exercise works on flexibility in the hip joint.

Crossover Figure Eights

Begin with your feet together, body in good alignment, stomach held in, and knees slightly bent. Keeping your toes pointed straight ahead, bend your out-

Bent-knee side leg swing

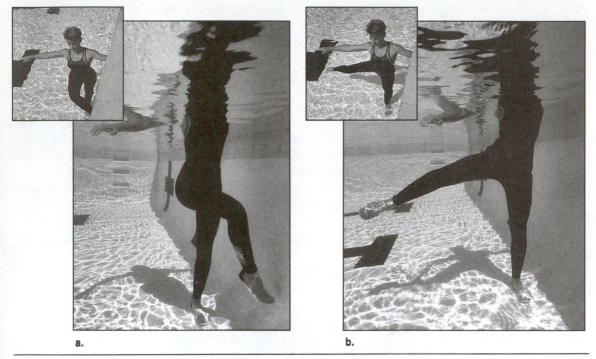

a.   b.

side leg at the knee (the one farthest from the side of the pool) and turn it out. Point your toe toward the floor of the pool. Keeping the knee bent throughout the movement, cross the knee in front of and beyond the supporting leg so that it moves toward the side of the pool. Turn the knee over and return it to the starting position. Complete the movement by leaving the knee in place and straightening the leg out to the side. Keep the toe pointed throughout the movement. Repeat the movement, but cross the bent knee behind the supporting leg. Crossing the working leg in front of and behind the supporting leg equals one repetition. Perform 10 to 15 repetitions to make one set, and execute one to four sets on each leg. Keep the movement smooth. Think of using your foot to describe a figure eight in the water with the foot in front and in back of the supporting leg on each repetition.

Caution

It is important to keep the supporting leg slightly bent and the body in good alignment throughout the exercise.

This exercise strengthens the waist (internal and external oblique), the inner thigh (adductors magnus, brevis and longus; gracilis, pectineus), and the outer thigh (tensor fascia lata). It also works the upper hip (gluteus medius and minimis).

Crossover figure eight

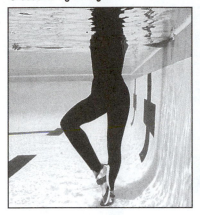

a.

b.

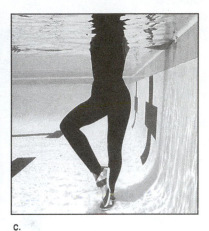

c.

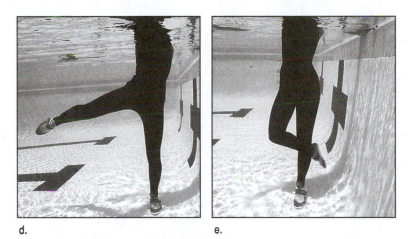

d.

e.

Leg Lift Back

Stand facing the side of the pool, with your hands on the edge. Begin with your feet together, body in good alignment, stomach held in, and knees slightly bent. Bend and lift your left leg up toward the surface of the water. Push the foot down and through the water to extend it straight behind you. Contract the buttock muscle as you push and lift the leg. Be sure to keep your back straight and your abdominal muscles pulled in and up to avoid arching your back. Do not lift the leg very high behind you. Perform 10 to 15 repetitions, or one set, on the left leg before changing to exercise the right leg. Execute one to four sets on each leg.

This exercise strengthens the buttocks (gluteus maximus) and the upper back of the thighs (hamstrings).

Leg lift back

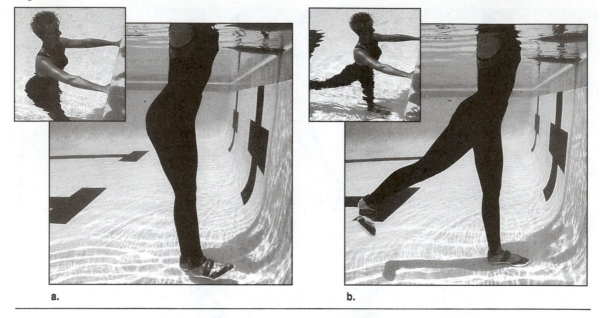

a.   b.

Abdominal Exercises

Knee Roll and Twists

Begin by placing your back up against the side wall of the pool. Extend your arms to the sides and hold on to the edge of the pool for support. Bend and pull your knees in toward your chest. (Your body will be suspended and supported by the water.) Keeping your knees together, roll them to a diagonal, pointing left. Keep your thighs, knees, and feet together. Now reverse the movement, and roll your thighs toward the right diagonal. Throughout the movement pull your abdominal muscles in and up and press your back and hips into the wall as much as possible.

Variation 1: Move away from the side wall of the pool, and support yourself holding a dumbbell-type flotation device in each hand instead of leaning on the wall.

Variation 2: At the completion of the roll to the diagonal position, extend your legs before bending them in and rolling to the other side.

This exercise strengthens the lower abdominal muscles (internal oblique and rectus abdominis).

Knees In and Out

Begin by placing your back up against the side wall of the pool, as you did in the previous exercise. Extend your arms to the sides, hold on to the edge of the pool for support, and suspend your body. Bend and pull your knees in toward your chest. Keeping your toes pointed and your legs together, straighten your legs in front of your body, trying to keep them near the surface of the water. Throughout the movement pull your abdominal muscles in and up and press

Knee roll and twist

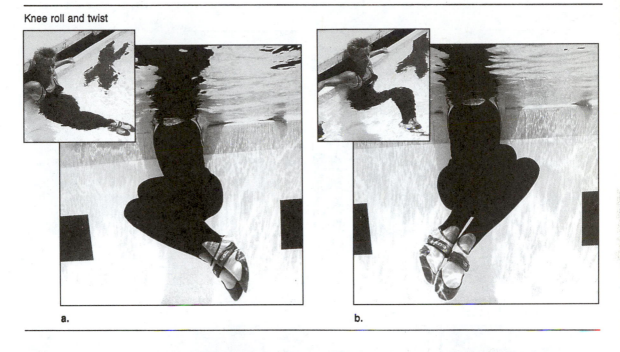

a.

b.

Knee roll and twist
with dumbbells

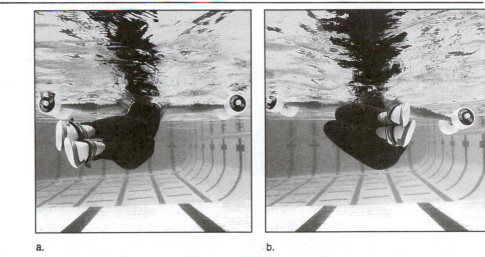

a.

b.

your back and hips into the wall as much as possible. Repeat 10 to 15 to complete one set, and execute one to four sets.

This exercise strengthens the lower abdominal muscles (internal oblique, rectus abdominis), the front of the thighs (quadriceps femoris group), and the upper front of the hip flexor area (iliopsoas).

Pull Knees In and Roll Through

Support yourself with a dumbbell-type flotation device in each hand. Keeping your body upright, pull your knees in toward your chest while contracting the

Knees in and out

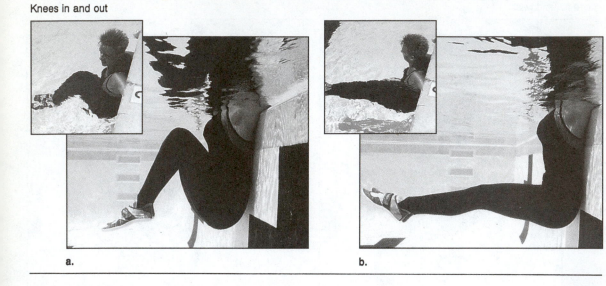

a.   b.

Pull knees in and roll through

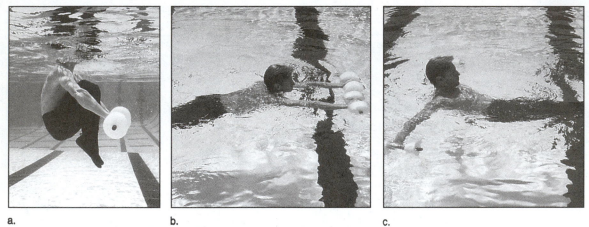

a.   b.   c.

abdominals throughout the movement. Then, keeping your knees tucked to your chest, gradually roll through onto your stomach to extend your legs behind you, almost parallel to the surface of the water. Your body will lean forward in the water. Reverse the movement. Repeat several times and gradually increase the repetitions.

Caution

Be careful not to hyperextend (arch) the lumbar (lower) area of your spine when you are on your stomach. Keep your abdominal muscles tucked in and tight throughout the movement so as not to place stress on your back. Move in a slow and controlled manner throughout the exercise.

This exercise strengthens the abdominal muscles (internal oblique, rectus abdominis), the front of the thighs (quadriceps femoris group), the upper front of the hip flexor area (iliopsoas), and the lower back (lumbar region).

Pedalling

Begin by placing your back up against the side wall of the pool, as you did in the previous exercises. Extend your arms to the sides and hold on to the edge of the pool for support. Bend and pull your knees in toward your chest. Pretend you are riding a bike while in this position and pedal your legs forward and backwards. Extend the movements all the way through the pushing action of your feet. Concentrate on holding your abdominal muscles in throughout the movements.

Variation 1: Support your body in the water using dumbbell-type flotation devices and execute the pedalling exercise while moving through the water.

Variation 2: Lean your body onto one side and pedal, which will move you in a circle, then reverse the direction.

This exercise strengthens the abdominal muscles (internal oblique, rectus abdominis), the front of the thighs (quadriceps femoris group), the upper front of the hip flexor area (iliopsoas), and the gluteal muscles.

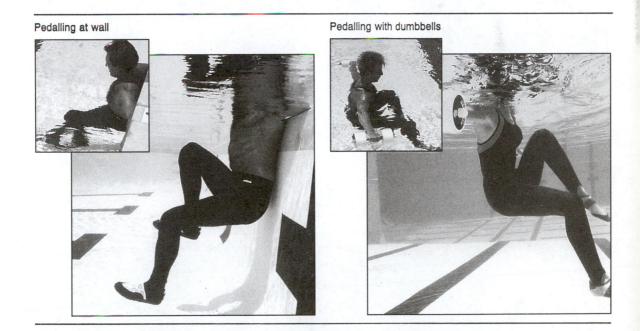

Pedalling at wall   Pedalling with dumbbells

Criss-Cross Scissors

Begin by placing your back up against the side wall of the pool for support, as you did in previous exercises. Extend your arms to the sides and grip the edge of the pool. Your body will be suspended with your back near or on the wall. Extend your legs in front of you so they are just below the surface of the water at a 90° angle to the hips. Begin with your legs together, straight, and toes pointed. Open your legs to each side, pushing the outside of your legs through the water to do so. Then squeeze your legs together, but allow the right leg to cross over slightly at the ankles when they are together. Repeat the movement, but this time let the left leg cross over the right at the ankles when they come together. Keep the movement smooth and continuous, and breathe steadily throughout the exercise. During the movement pull your abdominal muscles in and up and press your back and hips into the wall as much as possible. Completing one crossover with each leg equals one repetition. Perform 10 to 15 repetitions per set, and execute one to four sets.

Variation: This exercise can also be performed by using dumbbell-type flotation devices to support yourself in the water, away from the side of the pool.

This exercise strengthens the abdominal area (internal and external oblique, rectus abdominis), the inner thigh (adductors magnus, brevis, and longus; gracilis; pectineus), and the outer thigh (abductors and tensor fascia lata).

Criss-cross scissors

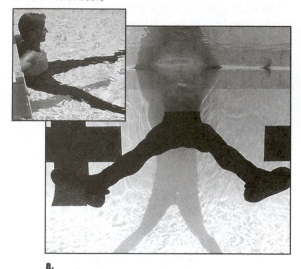
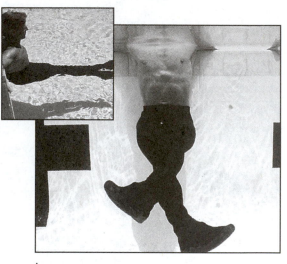

a.   b.

Criss-cross scissors with dumbbells

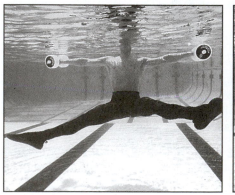
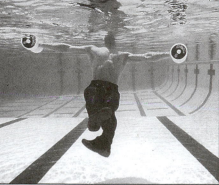

a.   b.

Calf and Ankle Exercise

Relevés or Ankle Raises

Stand on a step in the pool or on the edge and allow your heels to lower over the step (or edge). Hold on to the ladder for support. Keeping your body in good alignment with the abdominal muscles pulled in and standing upright, relevé or slowly raise yourself up onto the balls of your feet. Your legs should be straight, but do not lock your knees. Slowly and smoothly lower yourself to the starting position. Repeat 10 to 15 times to complete one set. Execute one to three sets.

This exercise strengthens the calf muscles (gastrocnemius and soleus) and shapes the legs.

Relevé (ankle raise)

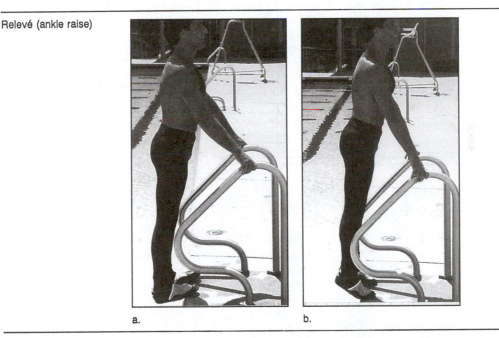

a.   b.

Stretches

This section includes a variety of stretching activities to be performed during the body of the class. These stretches will elongate the muscles contracted during your vigorous aerobic workout. As was mentioned earlier in this chapter, stretching should be performed after the body is fully warmed up, to increase flexibility. Use a sustained stretching technique when executing each movement. Ballistic movements or bouncing can cause injury to the body and do not promote flexibility. Be careful not to stretch to the point of pain or discomfort, but just to the point where you feel mild tension.

Side Stretch

Perform this side stretch in waist-deep water or on the pool deck. Stand sideways to the edge/side of the pool and place one hand on the pool's edge or a support on the deck. Extend your other arm to your side at shoulder height. Stretch your extended arm to the side and then overhead. Continue the stretch by allowing your hip to pull away from the pool's edge or the supporting structure. Hold this stretch for 10 seconds. Turn around and repeat on the other side. Repeat the entire exercise one or two more times on each side.

Side stretch

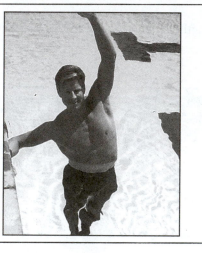

Hamstring Stretch

Stand in chest-deep water. Lift your right knee to your chest and hold your leg up under your knee. Keeping your back upright and straight, hold this stretch for 15 to 20 seconds. Alternate legs.

This exercise will stretch your hamstring muscles and your lower back.

Quadriceps Stretch

Stand sideways to the edge/side of the pool and place your right hand on the pool's edge. Bend your left knee, keeping it close to your right knee. With your left hand, gently lift the top of your left foot up so that your left sole moves toward your buttock. Hold the gentle stretch for 15 to 20 seconds. Turn around and stretch the other side in the same manner. Repeat. Remember to keep your body upright and in good alignment throughout the movement.

This exercise will stretch your quadriceps muscles.

Calf Stretch

Stand on a step in the pool, or the edge, and allow your right heel to lower over the edge. Hold on to the ladder for support if possible. Keeping your body in good alignment, standing upright and with the abdominal muscles pulled in, allow yourself to hold the stretch for 20 to 30 seconds. While stretching, be

Hamstring stretch   Quadriceps stretch

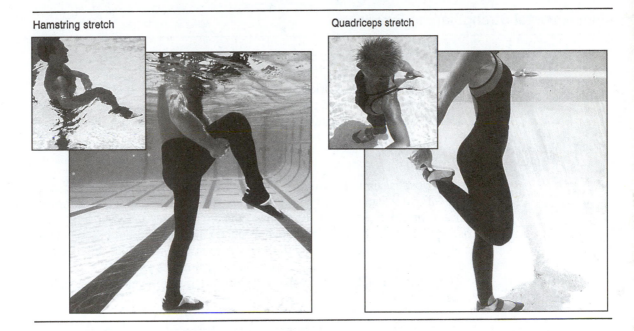

careful not to hyperextend your knee. Change sides and repeat the stretch.
Repeat the entire exercise again. This exercise will stretch the gastrocnemius
and soleus muscles used during the aerobic portion of your aqua aerobics class.

Shoulder and Leg Stretch

Stand with your back lightly touching the side of the pool for support. Contract
your abdominal muscles. Lift a bent right knee up toward the chest. Place your
left hand on the instep or toes of your right foot. Extend your right leg forward
and lift it up gently, as high as your body will let you. This action will stretch the
right hamstrings and the left shoulder area. Hold the stretch for 10 seconds.
Reverse onto the other side.

Calf stretch

Supplemental Strengthening Exercises

The following exercises can be used to supplement your aqua aerobics class. Some instructors include in-water exercises during their classes that will strengthen the muscles worked in the following exercises, and others don't. Use your own judgment if you would like to supplement the activities presented in class with these out-of-water exercises.

Push-Ups

Perform your maximum number of push-ups. Begin by lying on the floor, face down, with your fingers facing forward. Keep your feet together, your abdomen tight and pulled up, your weight on the balls of your feet, and your body in a straight line. Push yourself up until your elbows are straight, but not hyperextended. Lower your body halfway to the floor (to the point of a 90° angle at the elbows) to perform one push-up. Repeat as many times as you can.

This exercise will strengthen your shoulder girdle, pectoralis muscles, biceps, and triceps.

Note

Until you build up the upper-body strength to perform full-length push-ups, you may need to perform bent-knee push-ups. The upper-body performance is the same as just described; however, the weight of the lower body is supported on the tops of the knees.

Push-up

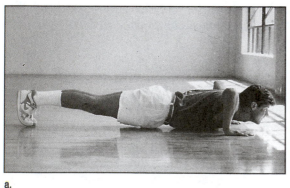

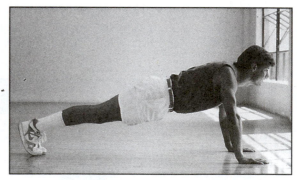

a.   b.

Reverse Push-Ups

This exercise strengthens your triceps muscles. Begin with your weight supported on your hands and feet and your back parallel to the floor. Your fingers must point toward your heels. Shift most of your weight toward your shoulders. Lower your body halfway to the floor, and then straighten your elbows to return to the starting position. Repeat as many times as possible.

Reverse push-up

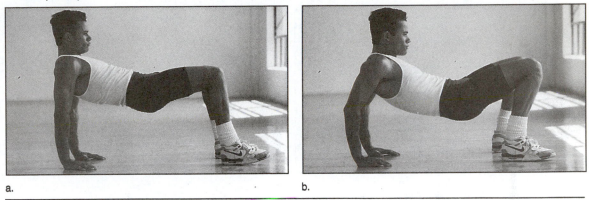

a.   b.

Abdominal Curl-Ups

Lie on your back with your knees bent and your feet flat. Place your right hand across your chest, on your left shoulder, and your left hand on your right shoulder. Lift your torso up halfway, keep your chin tucked toward your chest, and lift your head and shoulders off the floor. (If this hurts your neck, place your arms behind your head, touching opposite shoulders to cradle the head, and keep your eyes focused above you.) Exhale, contract your abdominal muscles, and press your lower back to the floor as you curl up. Release the contraction. Lower yourself to the floor one vertebrae at a time, being careful not to arch your back. Repeat the curl-up action as many times as you can.

Modifications for the Pregnant Exerciser. A good alternative to abdominal curls is to get on all fours and gently pull the abdomen in and contract while exhaling. Make sure the back does not arch. In advanced pregnancy, modify the abdominal work so that you roll back from an upright seated position to a backward lean of only 45°. However, this movement primarily works the hip flexor, and the abdominals run a distant second. (Chapter 9 discusses pregnancy and exercise in more detail.)

Abdominal curl-up

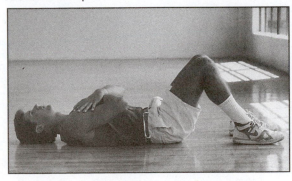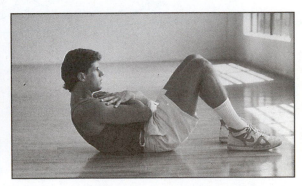

a.   b.

Abdominal contraction for pregnant exerciser

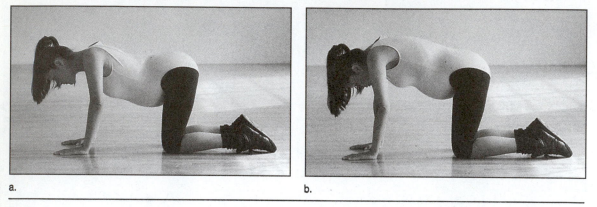

a.

b.

Kegels

Muscles of the pelvic floor are not usually exercised in a regular aqua aerobics class. Responsible for supporting the pelvic organs, these muscles hold the uterus floor in place and can prevent urinary incontinence and sexual dissatisfaction in women. The Kegel exercise, which strengthens these muscles located between the pubic bone in front and the coccyx in the back, should be emphasized for all women, but for the pregnant exerciser in particular. You can do this "invisible" little exercise by imagining that the area at the base of your pubic region is like an elevator floor. When you contract the correct muscles the elevator floor rises a few inches. These are the same muscles you use when you try to stop the flow of urine. Kegels should be done throughout a woman's lifetime, and particularly during pregnancy.

Body Area and Muscles Used During Activity

Exercise (Common Name)	Body Area; Muscles Used
Overhead and side stretches	Side of body; includes all muscles down the side of the body: external obliques, some involvement of latissimus dorsi, deltoids, serratus anterior, erector spinae.
Head isolation	Warms up neck muscles; includes trapezius and sternocleidomastoid.
Shoulder circles	Warms up entire shoulder area; deltoids, trapezius, latissimus dorsi, and serratus anterior.
Back warm-up	Muscles up the back; erector spinae, latissimus dorsi, rhomboideus, and abdominals.
Triceps stretch	Back of the arm; triceps and involvement of deltoids and trapezius.
Quadriceps stretch	Front of thighs; quadriceps and front of foot.
Calf stretches	Calf area, back of knee, lower leg, and back of ankle; gastrocnemius, soleus, and Achilles tendon.
Groin stretch	Inside of upper leg and back of leg at upper attachment; adductors and minor involvement of hamstrings.
Abductor stretch	Muscles on outer part of upper thigh and abdominals; abductor muscles and involvement of obliques.
Ankle raises	Tendon behind ankle, calf muscles, and minor involvement of buttocks and front of thighs; Achilles tendon, gastrocnemius, soleus, and minor involvement of gluteal muscles and quadriceps.
Heel walking	Strengthens front of lower leg and stretches calf muscles and back of

Exercise (Common Name)	Body Area; Muscles Used
	ankle; strengthens tibialis muscles and stretches gastrocnemius, soleus, and Achilles tendon.

Caution

Abdominal muscles and erector spinae are involved in all of the following. You need to concentrate on holding in your abdominal muscles throughout your movements.

Exercise (Common Name)	Body Area; Muscles Used
Walking; lunging; jogging; leaping; jumping; running; mountain climber; pony; rocking horse; slides; gallops; step, hop	Works entire front and back of legs as well as hip flexor and feet; also strengthens abdominal muscles when they are held in.
Twisting	Uses muscles involved in jumping as well as involves obliques, front and backs of arms, pectoralis, and shoulder area.
Frog leap; pendulum; step,hop; grapevine; schottische; grapevine schottische; jumping jacks	Works muscles on inside and outside of thighs, muscles at upper thigh–hip area, front of legs and feet, calf muscles, and some buttocks work; abductors, adductors, as well as hip flexor and entire quadriceps, tibialis, plantar flexor, gastrocnemius, soleus, with some involvement of gluteal muscles.
Echappé; hop, push foot; jack and boogie woogie; heel jack	Works inside and outside of upper thighs, front of legs and feet, buttocks muscles, and a little of the back of the legs; abductors, adductors, gastrocnemius, soleus, tibialis, as well as quadriceps, plantar flexor, and gluteal muscles, with minor involvement of hamstrings.
Hop, touch elbow to knee; can-can kick; hop, kick, and touch foot; jump, kick, and clap; charleston bounce step	Works upper front of thighs, torso and stomach areas, and fronts and backs of legs and feet; hip flexor, hamstrings, entire quadriceps, tibialis, and plantar flexor, gastrocnemius, soleus, rectus abdominis, and obliques.

Exercise (Common Name)	Body Area; Muscles Used
Breast stroke—arms	Works chest area, front and back of arms, shoulders and upper back; involves pectorals, deltoids, rhomboids, latissimus dorsi, biceps, triceps, and the muscles of the forearms.
Arm flies	Works chest area, front and back of arms, shoulders, and upper and middle back; pectorals, biceps, triceps, deltoids, trapezius, and rhomboids.
Biceps and triceps press	Works entire front and back of arms; triceps, biceps, and radialis.
Roller	Works front and backs of arms; biceps, triceps, brachialis, and forearm muscles.
Wall push-ups	Works arms, chest, back, and stomach areas; pectorals, biceps, triceps, abdominals, and erector spinae.
Press-ups	Works chest, shoulders, and back of arms; pectorals, trapezius, deltoids, and triceps.
Pectoral presses	Works chest, arms, shoulders, and back; pectorals, biceps, deltoids, trapezius, latissimus dorsi, rhomboids, and erector spinae.
Side leg lifts; bent-knee side leg lifts	Works inside and outside of upper thigh; abductors and adductors.
Side leg lift crossovers; crossover figure eights	Works inside and outside of upper thighs, front of hip at upper thigh, front of thighs, and buttocks muscles; abductors, adductors, hip flexor, quadriceps, and gluteal muscles.
Leg lift back	Works buttocks and back of upper thigh; gluteals and hamstrings.
Knee roll and twists; knees in and out	Works muscles in entire stomach area; lower abdominals, rectus abdominis, and obliques.
Pull knees in and roll through; pedalling	Works entire stomach area, front of hip area, front of thighs, and back;

Exercise (Common Name)	Body Area; Muscles Used
	lower abdominals, obliques, rectus abdominis, iliopsoas hip flexor, quadriceps, and erector spinae
Criss-cross scissors	Works inside and outside of upper thighs and stomach muscles; abductors, adductors, and abdominals.

Checklist: Your Personal Workout

I plan to work out:

_____ times per week in aqua aerobics class

_____ times per week participating in other activities

List activities:

_____

_____

_____

Directions: Record the date, activity, duration, and intensity (based on target heart rate) of your workout.

Date	Activity	Duration	Intensity (THR)
Example: 7/14	Tennis	30 minutes	140

Checklist: Stretch Workout

Directions: Write the date and check off the exercises you perform before class, after class, or on alternate days. Notate with a B for before class, an A for after class, and ALT for alternate-day exercising.

Exercise	Date	Number of Reps. and Sets	B, A, ALT
Overhead stretches			
Overhead side stretches			
Head isolations			
Shoulder circles			
Back stretches			
Quadriceps stretches			
Calf stretches			
Ankle circles			
Ankle raises			
Heel walking			
Other (list)			

Checklist: Supplemental Strengthening Exercises

Directions: Record below the dates you perform the exercises listed and whether they have been done after class or on alternate days. Notate with an A for after class or ALT for alternate-day exercising.

Exercise	Date	Number of Reps. and Sets	A, ALT
Push-ups			
Reverse push-ups			
Abdominal curl-ups			
Other (list)			

Summary

1. Most aquatic exercise instructors begin a class with warm-up activities and gentle stretches in the pool.
2. Exercise physiologists have demonstrated that flexibility as a result of stretching will only increase if the muscles are warm.
3. Remember never to use ballistic or jerky stretches—all stretching movements should be smooth and sustained.
4. You need to allow yourself nine to fifteen minutes for a good overall body warm-up.
5. The first three to five minutes of a warm-up in the pool is called a *thermal warm-up*. Its main purpose is to warm up the major muscles, which will allow the body to deliver extra oxygen to the working muscle tissues.

   The *pre-stretch* section of the warm-up allows time for you to execute mild stretches for body parts you will be using in the cardiovascular workout (i.e., groin, lower back, ankles, shoulders, etc.).

   The *cardiovascular warm-up* period is the time when you begin to place stress on the cardiovascular system by slowly jogging in place or walking/running through the water to prepare your body for the upcoming 20- to 40-minute aerobic workout.
6. A nine- to fifteen-minute in-pool warm-up is advised before beginning strenuous aerobic activities. The warm-up is divided as follows:

Thermal warm-up	Three to five minutes.
Pre-stretch	Three to five minutes.
Cardiovascular warm-up	Three to five minutes.

7. A 20- to 40- minute aerobic section follows the warm-up period.
8. A 10- to 15-minute cool-down, including stretching and strengthening movements, follows.
9. When performing the exercises described in this chapter, use the best possible body alignment to gain the most benefit from each exercise and to avoid injuries.
10. Land-based strengthening exercises can be used to supplement your aqua aerobics class.

CHAPTER 8

Choreographing Your Own Aqua Aerobics Routines

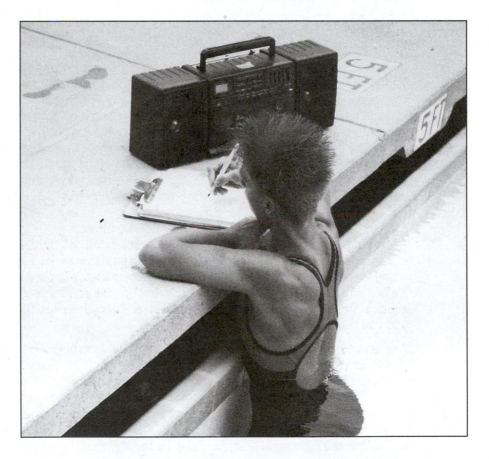

Outline

Many students like to create (choreograph) their own aquatic exercise routines to music that they enjoy. Choreographing your own routines can be very creative and satisfying. Keep in mind that the choreographic goal of aqua aerobics is to coordinate to music combined patterns of movement and often dance steps, in the water, that keep you moving continuously so you can exercise your body and, in turn, your heart. The aerobic portion of the workout should be 20 to 30 minutes long, allowing you to reach and work at your target heart rate and thus giving you the exercise training effect that you desire.

Creating Your Aquatic Aerobics Routine

First, select your music. The music should have a steady beat as well as a motivating, upbeat feeling that makes you want to work hard. The tempo should be approximately 120 to 140 beats per minute. Once you select your music, listen to it and analyze the musical phrasing. Usually the music is composed such that you can create phrases of movement (movement sequences) that take eight counts. You can create several phrases of eight counts of movement and then combine them in various ways to fit the composition of the music. Each phrase you create can be given a letter to identify it. If you create four phrases, letter them A, B, C, and D. Then combine the phrases in any order you like; for example, A B C D A B A B C D. The phrases can be repeated in any order, and as many times as you want, as long as they fit with the music.

You don't have to be a dancer to create a well-balanced, enjoyable, high-energy routine. While creating your routine, pay attention to the fact that you want to work the muscles in your body in a balanced way. Work opposing muscles of a pair (such as biceps and triceps, quadriceps and hamstrings, etc.) equally. An example of four phrases of movement (identified as A, B, C, and D) that you could combine into a routine are:

A: Perform eight running with arm scoops movements in place.
B: Perform four cat leaps to the right and then four cat leaps to the left.
C: Beginning on your right foot, perform four rocking horse movements by traveling forward and using front-crawl-type arm movements, and then swing your left leg through to the front and perform four rocking horse movements with the same arms on your left side.
D: Slide to the right eight times, and clap on the eighth slide. While sliding, begin with the arms to the sides, then move both arms simultaneously in a scooping action. Repeat the movement phrase to the left.

These phrases can be first performed in the A B C D format and then combined in any order you feel works well with the music. A simple way to add variety is to do different arm movements each time you repeat the phrase or change the direction of the movement. When you make a variation, identify that lettered phrase with a subscript number. For example, let's say the original phrase is lettered A. The next time you repeat A vary the arm movements and identify that specific phrase as A_1. Your new routine might be: A B C D A_1 B_1 C_1 D_1 A B C D. In this routine, you use the original four phrases, change the arm movements that accompany each phrase, and then repeat the original four phrases of movement.

More challenging and diversified routines use more than four phrases in combination. It is up to you how many phrases you would like to create and use in each routine. Movement phrases longer than eight counts may be difficult for you to remember at the beginning. However, when you become more experienced you can challenge yourself by creating longer routines and utilizing more complex movements. You can also write your own routines on paper, encase them in plastic, and keep them on the side of the pool.

The phrases you use in your aqua aerobics routines are only limited by your abilities and creativity. You can use all of the aerobic movements listed in Chapter 7 as basic movement patterns, combined in any order, as well as movements you invent for the creation of your routines. The aerobic movements described in Chapter 7 are representative of the types of steps you can use; there is really no limit to the phrases you can create. So have fun and make up routines to which you would like to exercise!

Caution
_____

Remember to use proper body alignment and a variety of muscle groups when creating movements and movement phrases.

Once you have choreographed the aerobic portion of your workout you will then need to select movements for the pre-class warm-up section, the in-pool aqua aerobic activities section (which will include your choreographed activities), the upper-body strengthening and toning section, the legwork exercise section, the abdominal exercise section, and the supplemental strengthening exercise section to put together an entire aqua aerobics workout that you can execute outside of class.

Sample Eight-Count Phrases of Movement

(See Chapter 7 for a more complete listing of movements and their descriptions.) The following are examples of movement phrases that can be used during the aerobics section of your workout. Remember to perform a nine- to fifteen-minute warm-up before beginning this section of movement.

- Jog in place eight times, using front-crawl-type arm movements in coordination with each jog.
- Jog in place while scooping your arms from side to side, parallel to the water's surface.
- Run in place eight times while lifting your feet toward your buttocks in the rear. Use pumping-type arm movements.
- Hop and kick in place eight times, alternating your legs and pushing down and through the water in opposition to each leg movement.
- Perform eight jumping jacks, moving your arms down and up (to shoulder level) in coordination with the leg movements.
- Mountain climber: With your feet separated, jump and land forward and backward a distance of about one foot. Alternate feet as you land in front and in back on each jump. Your arms can push through the water in opposition to the leg movements.
- Pony (hop, step, step): Hop on the right foot to the side, then quickly step with the left foot and then the right foot. Repeat on the other side. Make

double-scooping arm movements at chest level, one large scoop per pony phrase (hop, step, step).

- Slide four times to the right and then slide four times to the left. Repeat several times.
- Hop on one foot and lift up the opposite knee. The opposite elbow approaches the opposite knee on a diagonal plane. Keep the back upright during the movement. Reverse and repeat eight times.
- Hop on one foot, and swing kick the opposite foot forward and then to the back. The arms move in opposition, pressing through the water. Reverse and repeat eight times.
- Charleston bounce step: Use a very bouncy step throughout this phrase. Step right, kick the left foot forward, step back on the left foot, and touch the right toe back. Repeat two times (eight counts). The arms move in opposition to the kicking leg and press through the water forward and backward in coordination with the leg movements.
- Can-can kick: Hop on the right foot, and simultaneously bring the bent left knee up to a 90° angle in front. Hop again on the right foot and kick the left foot through the water in front of the body. Try to extend the left leg straight out at a 90° angle. Repeat four times, and then do the sequence on the other side. A more advanced version involves alternating sides after each kick.
- Schottische: Run three times in place or while traveling forward through the water and then hop and clap simultaneously (run R, L, R, hop R). Alternate sides four times.
- Grapevine: While traveling to the right, step to the right, cross your left foot behind the right foot and step on the left, step to the right on the right foot, cross the left foot in front of the right foot, and step on the left foot while traveling to the right. Repeat this phrase two times, moving to the right. To perform the grapevine in reverse with a smooth transition, begin by stepping on the left foot to the left before crossing the right foot behind the left foot.
- Grapevine schottische: Step to the right on the right foot, cross the left foot behind the right foot, step on the right foot to the right, and hop on the right foot. To reverse, step on the left foot to the left, cross the right foot behind the left foot and step on it, step on the left foot to the left, and hop on the left foot. Repeat.
- Run three times in place, and kick and clap on the fourth count. Alternate sides. Repeat the phrase four times.
- Twist the body while using a bounce landing, and swing the arms in opposition overhead or at chest level on each twist.
- Jump kick: Jump and kick the right foot forward, and then jump and kick the left foot forward. Vary the movement by kicking the leg on a diagonal and alternating the direction of the kick. Perform four jump kicks, alternating sides. The arms push through the water in opposition to the leg movements.
- Skier's jump: Jump to the right while twisting the body toward the left diagonal. Reverse on the other side. Perform eight times. For variety, you can jump twice on each side before changing directions. (Jumping twice takes two counts; therefore, only perform four.) The arms scoop simultaneously in front of the body, moving in the opposite direction of the skier's jump.

Samples of Routines Choreographed to Music

Following are two sample routines to be used in the aerobic section of your workout. The purpose of describing these routines is twofold:

1. To provide you with routines that you can perform to the pieces of music selected, if you so choose; and
2. To demonstrate how a routine will look upon completion.

Glenn Miller Medley Routine*
(Music by Jive Bunny and the Master Mixers)

Introduction

During the musical introduction, twist with your arms moving through the water from side to side, chest high.

Part I

1. Jog forward four times.
2. Jumping jacks, moving backward four times.
3. Rocking horse (right, left, right, kick the left leg forward).
4. Rocking horse (left, right, left, kick the right leg forward).
5. Jump twist three times, then jump to a position where your feet are shoulder-width apart and then jump again.
6. Repeat Part I, 1-5.
7. Jog in place four times.

Part II

1. Leap to the right four times, leading with the right foot.
2. Rocking horse back right, front left, back right, turn body to the left.
3. Repeat the above two phrases, beginning to the left on the left foot.
4. Pendulum three times. Repeat four sets.
5. Leap to the right four times.
6. Leap to the left four times.
7. Jump and bounce in place two times.

Part III

1. Hop and kick eight times to the front, alternating legs on each hop and kick.
2. Hop and kick eight times, pointing the kicking leg toward each diagonal and alternating legs and diagonals.

Part IV

1. Support yourself on your left leg. Kick the right leg forward four times while pressing your arms, which should be extended to the sides at the surface of the water, backward.
2. Repeat the above phrase, kicking the right leg to the back while pressing the arms forward.
3. Step onto the right foot and simultaneously turn your body 90° to the right. Supporting yourself on your right leg, repeat the above phrase, now kicking forward and then backward with the left leg.

*Contributed by Julie See.

4. Step onto the left foot, turn 90° to the left, and repeat the phrase facing forward again.
5. Step onto the right foot, turn 90° to the left, and repeat the phrase facing the left side.
6. Step backward onto the right foot, turn 90° to the right, and repeat the phrase facing forward again.
7. Step backward onto the left foot, turn 90° to the right, and repeat the phrase facing the right side.

Part V

Jog eight times in a small circle to the right, pulling your arms through the water as in front crawl, half-time (R, L, R, L). (Half-time means to take two beats to complete each arm movement.)

Part VI

1. Rocking horse three times beginning forward on the right (R, L, R), then kick the left leg forward.
2. Jump twist three times. Repeat two sets.
3. Jog forward four times.
4. Jumping jacks backward four times.

Ending

Jog in a circle until the music ends. (If performing this routine with a group of people, jog into a circle, take each other's hands, and jog in the circle holding hands until the music ends.)

"Pink Cadillac" Routine*
(Music by Aretha Franklin)

Part I

1. Extend your right arm forward above the water (use a front-crawl armstroke) and press it down and backward through the water using eight beats of the music.
2. Repeat with the left arm.
3. Execute the above using both arms simultaneously.

Part II

Slide and shimmy: Slide to the right four times. On each slide, shimmy your shoulders while holding your arms extended to the side, just below or above the surface of the water. Repeat the phrase three times moving to the left, then the right, and finally the left again.

Part III

1. Slow walk to the right: Moving to the right, take a large step onto the right foot using two beats. Keep your head turned to the right side during the step. Drag and pull the left leg into the right and step onto the left foot. Simultaneously turn your head to the front. Use two beats to complete the drag-and-pull movement. Repeat the step, drag, and pull three times.

*Contributed by Julie See.

2. Repeat the entire phrase moving to the left.

Part IV

1. Jog in a box pattern: Slowly jog four times forward (R, L, R, L), taking two beats per jog. Lift the heels up to approach the buttocks on each jog. Turn 90° to the right and repeat the four jogs; again turn 90° to the right and repeat; and once more turn 90° to the right and repeat.
2. Repeat the jog in a box pattern beginning on the left foot and performing each 90° turn to the left.

Part V

Perform four jumping jacks.

Part VI

("Pink Cadillac" chorus—sing along). Side lunges and arm scoops: Lunge to the right onto the right leg and simultaneously scoop the right arm through the water, parallel to the surface, from the right side to the left side in front of the body. Take four beats to lunge and scoop the arm. Repeat to the left. Repeat until you have performed eight lunges, alternating sides. On the fifth lunge, lift your arms up and out of the water and wave when the music says "waving to the girls."

Part VII

Jog in place three times. Repeat three sets.

Part VIII

Jog in place eight times.

Part IX

Repeat Parts III, IV, V, VI, and VII.

Part X

Double knee lifts: Take four beats to perform each double knee lift—jump and pull both knees toward the chest. Perform a total of eight double knee lifts.

Part XI

Repeat Parts III, IV, V, VI, and VII.

Selecting Music to Create Your Own Routines

When creating your own routines, you need to decide what music to use. The simplest solution, of course, is to use music you already have. However, the tempo won't necessarily be appropriate for the exercises you want to do. Select music that motivates you and has a steady beat, approximately 120 to 140 beats per minute. The warm-up section needs the music at 120 beats per minute, the aerobic section may need up to 140 beats per minute, and the strengthening and cool-down sections will use approximately 120 beats per minute.

You can spend hours attempting to find the right music. Several companies sell music for aqua aerobics and aerobics; they have adjusted the tempo of contemporary songs to fit warm-up activities; aqua aerobics; aqua cool-down; and strength, flexibility, and stretching exercises. Several of the companies from which you can order music for aqua aerobics are listed in Appendix E. Music intended for low-impact classes and step/bench aerobics also can be used for aqua aerobics.

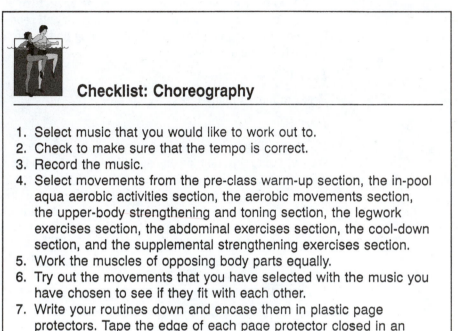

Checklist: Choreography

1. Select music that you would like to work out to.
2. Check to make sure that the tempo is correct.
3. Record the music.
4. Select movements from the pre-class warm-up section, the in-pool aqua aerobic activities section, the aerobic movements section, the upper-body strengthening and toning section, the legwork exercises section, the abdominal exercises section, the cool-down section, and the supplemental strengthening exercises section.
5. Work the muscles of opposing body parts equally.
6. Try out the movements that you have selected with the music you have chosen to see if they fit with each other.
7. Write your routines down and encase them in plastic page protectors. Tape the edge of each page protector closed in an attempt to waterproof your written routines.
8. Execute the post-class stretches.

Summary

1. Many students find choreographing routines to music they enjoy a creative experience.
2. The aqua aerobics routine you create should last 20 to 30 minutes and be strenuous enough to allow you to reach your target heart rate.
3. Select music that motivates you and has a steady beat, approximately 120 to 140 beats per minute.
4. Create movement phrases consisting of eight counts each. Label each phrase with a letter, such as A, B, C, and D. Then combine the lettered phrases in the pattern that they best fit the music, for example, A B C D A C D B A. There is no limit to the way you can combine your movements. Have fun!
5. Remember that you may want to monitor your heart rate or perceived exertion rate during and at the end of your aqua aerobics workout to see whether you are staying in your target heart rate zone or exceeding it. However, remember that there are many factors affecting it.

CHAPTER 9

Exercisers With Special Needs

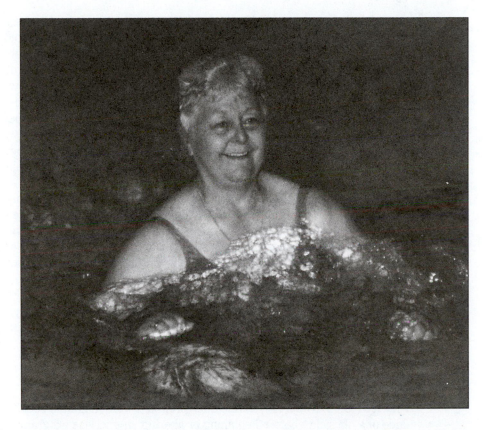

Outline

Exercisers with special needs that are temporary or permanent in nature will be discussed in this chapter. Such exercisers include those who are pregnant, obese, older, arthritic, asthmatic, physically challenged, or who have joint pain, cardiac problems, or temporary or chronic injuries.

Pregnancy and Exercise

Value

Pregnancy and aqua aerobics can be safe partners. Aqua aerobics can have a healthy and positive effect on a mother-to-be, and help her with a rapid recovery during the post-partum period. Exercise done during pregnancy should be cleared through an obstetrician prior to beginning. The general rule of thumb for a pregnant woman with an uncomplicated pregnancy is that if she was exercising before she became pregnant then it's all right to continue exercising during the pregnancy. Also, women who have been sedentary before becoming pregnant are encouraged to exercise during pregnancy; however, it would be unwise suddenly to take up such strenuous activities as weight training, skiing, or horseback riding if you hadn't done those activities prior to becoming pregnant.

Exercising during pregnancy does not necessarily decrease labor time or ensure a healthier baby. It does, however, provide many benefits to the mother. Research supports the notion that the exercising mother-to-be can maintain her own cardiovascular fitness, musculoskeletal strength, and flexibility. Benefits to the fetus are unknown; but there are sufficient data to support the theory that the fetus is not endangered during a pregnant woman's consistent exercise for periods of 15 minutes or less when her heart rate is no higher than 140 beats per minute. As the pregnancy advances, the mother-to-be and her physician should continue to evaluate her tolerance to aerobic-type exercising and whether or not she should exercise to full term.

Special Precautions

Medical Clearance. As stated earlier, pregnant women should seek the clearance of a physician before beginning or altering an exercise program.

Fluids. Pregnant women are encouraged to drink water freely before, during, and after a workout to avoid dehydration. Exercise can raise the body's core temperature to dangerous levels that could pose a risk to fetal health, especially during the first three months of pregnancy.

Modifications of Aerobic Exercising for the Pregnant Exerciser

Important modifications of aerobic exercising need to be made for pregnant women. The following is a list of general modifications and guidelines adapted from both the American College of Obstetricians and Gynecologists (ACOG) and a symposium, lecture, and video course called *Pregnancy the Aerobic Way*, developed by Bonnie Rote, RN, a consultant to the American Fitness Association of America (AFAA), and Kenneth Sekine, MD.

Warm-Up. Due to the pregnant woman's increased risk of orthopedic injury, a warm-up of 10 to 12 minutes is the minimum time period recommended. Most aqua aerobics instructors do provide a warm-up period of at least 10 minutes. During pregnancy, estrogen and progesterone cause tissues and joints to soften and become unstable. When joints are unstable, ligaments and tendons are in greater danger of tears or strains. The enlarged breasts and uterus alter the center of gravity and produce a greater strain on the lower back. An increased load is also placed on the sacroiliac and hip joints, which can feel like a sore tailbone at times. Working out in water, however, helps support the body and thus less strain is placed on the woman while doing aqua aerobics than if she were engaging in other forms of aerobic exercising. It is fatiguing for pregnant exercisers to maintain proper body alignment while standing on land. However, in aqua aerobics the water helps support the body, and proper alignment can more easily be maintained.

Smooth, controlled, static stretches are essential to a proper warm-up. Static stretches for the hamstring, inner thigh, and calf can all be performed in the water safely, smoothly, and rhythmically. Ballistic movements should never be performed during warm-up or cool-down.

Rhythmic limbering is the second essential element to a proper warm-up for all exercisers, but particularly for pregnant women. Walking in the shallow water as well as rhythmic upper-body movements are good warm-up exercises.

Cardiovascular Work. During pregnancy, the mother-to-be's blood volume increases by 50 percent. This diluted volume results in a lower oxygen-carrying capacity, which reduces the cardiac reserve during physical activity. In addition, the expanding uterus reduces the size of the lung cavity, causing a mild hyperventilation during rest that does not increase proportionately with exercise. Because of these changes in the body, the time and intensity of the aerobic workout should be altered. Many pregnant women may be unable to maintain high levels of aerobic activity.

To adapt to aerobic work when pregnant, lower the target heart rate to 50 to 60 percent of maximum for beginners, gradually increasing to 70 percent of maximum for intermediate to advanced. It's wise to maintain a target heart rate of no higher than 65 percent during the final stages of pregnancy. The American College of Obstetricians and Gynecologists recommends never exceeding 140 beats per minute (see target heart rate calculations).

The amount of time spent in continuous aerobic movement should not exceed 15 minutes, according to ACOG. Use how you feel as a guideline for your workout. A useful measure is Borg's Perceived Exertion Scale (see the Perceived Exertion Rating Scale section in Chapter 2), since heart rate response itself may be variable and inconsistent.

Obese Exercisers

Many persons suffering from obesity feel similar to pregnant women when they try to exercise. The excess weight makes it difficult for them to feel comfortable exercising on land. Fortunately, since water supports 80 to 90 percent of their body weight, obese persons can comfortably exercise in water and improve their overall body condition. Another advantage of exercising in water is that since the majority of the body is submerged under water no one can see the exerciser's body, which should allow a person who may be sensitive about his/her body to feel less uncomfortable.

Obese and pregnant exercisers are often self-conscious about their bodies when walking to the pool or exercise area. A simple solution is to use some sort of a cover-up; for example, a t-shirt, large towel, terry cloth robe, or shorts.

Arthritis, Joint Pain, Chronic Injuries, and Injury Rehabilitation

Other populations that need to be addressed in this chapter are people with arthritis, joint pain, chronic injuries, and those undergoing injury rehabilitation. The aquatic environment offers a wonderful area in which to exercise when, for one reason or another, your joints aren't in their best condition.

Research indicates that exercise makes it possible for those with arthritis to manage their lives with more independence and less pain. There are several types of arthritis that benefit from aquatic exercise. They are:

1. *Hypertrophic*, also know as osteo-arthritis. This is a form of chronic arthritis occurring mainly in elderly people and marked by degeneration and hypertrophy of the bone and cartilage and thickening of the synovial membrane. Prior injuries can predispose a joint to osteo-arthritis.

2. *Rheumatoid*, a chronic disease of the joints, usually marked by inflammatory changes in the synovial membranes and degeneration of the bones. Deformation develops in the victim. This disease destroys both sides of the cartilage at a joint. Rheumatoid arthritis affects approximately 1 percent of the population.

3. *Vertebral*, which involves inflammation of the intervertebral disks.

4. *Acute gouty*, which is associated with gout.

These forms of arthritis are the most common, and gentle movement of affected joints, muscles, ligaments, and tendons through the water helps maintain their mobility. People suffering from arthritis benefit from keeping their joints mobile. The water provides the ideal cushioning environment to help individuals with arthritis stay fit.

Similarly, people recovering from injuries and needing rehabilitation can regain or maintain their muscular condition by exercising in an aquatic environment. The water supports the body and takes the weight and stress off the joints while the muscles are working to gain, regain, or maintain their physical condition. Additionally, the movement of the water around the body acts as a very mild massage and feels good. The exhilaration of the water allows people suffering from joint and muscular weakness, regardless of the cause, to feel better physically and emotionally after a water workout. It also helps their muscular and cardiovascular systems improve as a direct result of working out in the water. Often people recovering from an injury shy away from exercising when various parts of their body hurt, but with aquatic exercise everyone can work out and rehabilitate in a safe manner.

Older Exercisers

Aquatic exercisers come in all sizes, colors, shapes, and ages. There are 65-year-old exercisers in better overall physical condition than many 35-year-old exercisers. Age is not a factor that limits participation in aqua aerobics. Age may slow down some exercisers a little and their hearing and vision might not be as acute as those of a younger exerciser, but there really are no age limits for participants in aqua aerobics.

Checklist: Before You Begin an Exercise Program

The important considerations when embarking on an exercise program were discussed earlier in the textbook. Points worth repeating are:

1. If you have been sedentary, have a physical examination and discuss participation in an aquatic exercise program with your physician before you take your first class.
2. Participate in the class you've selected using personal caution and awareness—gradually increase the exercise intensity over a period of weeks.
3. Listen to your body's signals. Monitor your perceived exertion rate and your heart rate during and after your class.

Remember, age in and of itself is not a limiting factor—your health and your physical condition are. Use your years of life experience and common sense to guide you through safe participation in aqua aerobics.

Asthma

Asthma is a condition that causes the bronchial passages to the lungs to swell, thus reducing the airflow. An asthma victim will wheeze, cough, and, in serious attacks, gasp for breath. Prolonged attacks can be disabling or even fatal (although fatalities are rare). Asthma is caused by a variety of elements, including allergies, exercise, and emotions. Exercise-induced asthma is brought on when a susceptible individual is involved in aerobic-type activities. Persons with asthma can exercise with ease when they use the proper medications and are under the care of a physician. The warm, moist exercise environment associated with aqua aerobics is soothing to some individuals suffering from exercise-induced asthma, although others may not respond that way.

The Physically-Challenged Exerciser

Aquatic exercise is the perfect environment for persons who are physically challenged with a disability. The water helps support and balance the individual, and also provides resistance to the participant. Non-swimmers who are physically disabled need to use buoyancy apparatus and have an able-bodied partner to work one on one with them. Additionally, a lifeguard must be on duty whenever a physically disabled nonswimmer is exercising in the water.

Exercisers with partial paralysis of the side of the body or paralysis of an individual limb most likely can integrate easily into any aqua aerobics class. It may be necessary to place a flotation device on the weak body part(s); this should be discussed with the exerciser's physician and the instructor before beginning a program. Persons with more extensive paralysis may need to participate in adapted-type aquatic exercise classes offered at rehabilitation centers, hospitals, and public agencies such as the YWCA or YMCA.

Summary

1. In general, as long as a pregnant woman is in good health and has medical clearance from her physician, she can safely participate in an aqua aerobics class.
2. Due to the changing orthopedic structure of a pregnant woman's body, the warm-up period may need to be extended to ensure that the body is adequately prepared for exercising. Both rhythmic limbering and mild walking through water are good additional warm-up exercises.
3. During cardiovascular work, the pregnant exerciser is cautioned against exceeding a heart rate of 140 beats per minute or 65 percent of her maximum heart rate.
4. Exercises that irritate and stress the supporting ligaments should be avoided by pregnant exercisers.
5. Safety is the key factor for pregnant exercisers (as for all exercisers).
6. Most obese people feel better exercising in the water, as do most pregnant women, because the water helps support their body weight, which usually inhibits their ability to exercise aerobically on land.
7. Exercising in the water helps hide the body from the eyes of onlookers, allowing participants who feel inhibited or self-conscious to work out in an unrestrained manner.
8. Water exercise provides an environment ideal for people suffering from arthritis to maintain joint mobility.
9. Aquatic exercise allows persons needing muscular and joint rehabilitation, regardless of the cause, to feel exhilarated and to improve their muscular and cardiovascular condition.
10. Age in and of itself is not a factor that limits safe participation in aqua aerobics; health and physical condition are the more important factors affecting participation in aquatic exercise.
11. Individuals with asthma can safely participate in aqua aerobics when under a physician's care.
12. Aquatic exercise is the perfect exercise environment for persons who are physically challenged with a disability. The water helps support the individual and also provides resistance to him/her.

CHAPTER 10

Equipment and Aqua Aerobics

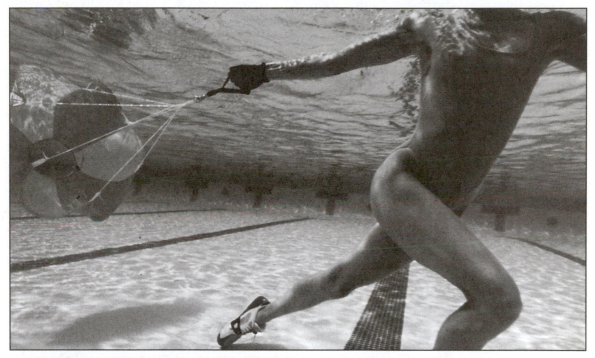

Wave Aerobics "Wave Chutes" designed by Mary Sanders.
Photo by Tracy Frankel for SHAPE Magazine, August, 1992.

Outline

Aqua aerobics classes, as described earlier in this textbook, are fun and complete on their own. However, your aquatic workout or aqua aerobics classes can be supplemented with a variety of equipment available on the market. The equipment adds variety to your workout, can contribute to it in a deep-water dimension, and can improve strength development, depending on the equipment selected. This equipment includes webbed gloves, water-supportive and water-resistant dumbbell-type buoys, flotation equipment for deep-water workouts, water-resistant equipment, and pull buoys. Most of the equipment is trademarked and offers types of workout activities specific to the equipment. Brief descriptions of some of the equipment available for use in your workouts follow. Sources for purchasing the equipment are listed in Appendix F of this textbook.

Hydro-Fit Equipment

Hydro-Fit equipment consists of buoyancy cuffs that can be worn on the ankles or around the waist, hand-held dumbbell-type buoys, and webbed water-resistance gloves. Hydro-Fit aquatic fitness equipment increases the surface area that is pushed or pulled through the water, thus enhancing the water's natural resistance quality; the use of this equipment increases your workout possibilities. The supportive cuffs allow for no-impact, deep-water cardiovascular and strengthening exercising. Using the equipment, the Hydro-Fit conditioning program consists of 10 lower-body movements, 12 arm exercises, 4 wall exercises, and 3 types of abdominal exercises.

Hydro-Tone Equipment

Another type of equipment available on the market that can greatly enhance the strength portion of your aquatics workout is Hydro-Tone equipment. The Hydro-Tone aquatic exercise system consists of water exercises enhanced by the use of Hydro-Bells held in the hands and Hydro-Boots worn on the feet. Using the equipment allows you to experience smooth, stable, three-dimensional resistance as you move the equipment through the water. The degree of the resistance varies with the effort applied. The use of Hydro-Tone equipment in aquatic exercising enhances muscle tone, strength, cardiovascular strength and endurance, flexibility, and body composition. The unique feature of the Hydro-Tone exercise equipment is the "accommodating variable resistance" phenomenon. According to James Counsilman, Ph.D., "The degree of resistance encountered depends upon the speed and direction at which the Hydro-Tone equipment is moved through the water: resistance is proportional to the square of the velocity of movement." Scientific analysis of this phenomenon is illustrated by the graph on page 155.

Hydro-Fit Exercises

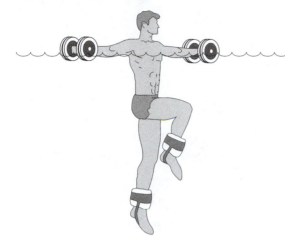

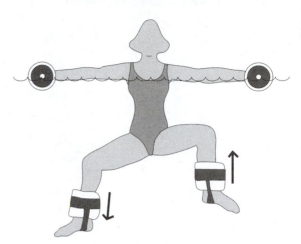

KNEE HIGH JOG

With body erect and legs straight, lift one knee toward your chest. As you straighten your leg to the starting position, lift your other knee toward your chest. Repeat. Strengthens and tones thighs and buttocks.
TIP: To increase intensity, increase speed.

TIRE PUMPS

With body erect and legs turned outward, lift your knee keeping your leg turned outward. Straighten your leg as you push down and outward. Repeat with other leg. Keep legs moving in a "pumping" action, as if running through tires. Strengthens and tones thighs, trunk, and buttocks.
TIP: Keep legs turned outward and feet flexed.

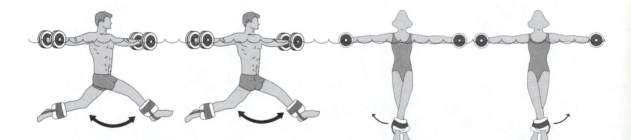

CROSS COUNTRY

With legs straight and body erect, extend one leg forward and one leg back. Swing your legs through the water front-to-back and back-to-front. Stabilize yourself by keeping buoys at the surface with arms held out to your sides. Strengthens and tones thighs, buttocks, trunk, and hip flexors.
TIP: For more resistance, keep knees straight and toes pointed.

SCISSORS

With body erect and legs straight, lift legs shoulder distance apart. Bring legs together in a scissoring motion, alternating the front leg. Stabilize yourself by keeping buoys at the surface with arms held out to your sides. Strengthens and tones buttocks and thighs.
TIP: Begin with 10-15 reps, increase to 30-60 reps.

Hydro-Fit Exercises (continued)

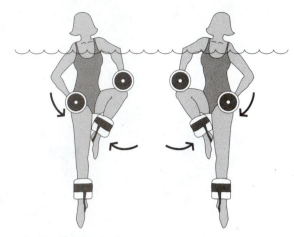

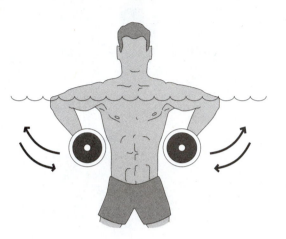

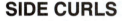

CUFF TOUCH

With body erect and legs straight, lift arms away from sides, keeping elbows bent. Bend at the waist and alternate touching left buoy to right foot and right buoy to left foot. Strengthens and tones chest, trunk, and thighs.

TIP: Concentrate on using your abdominal muscles.

SIDE CURLS

With bouys at the surface and arms held out to your sides, bend elbows and pull buoys into sides. Return arms to starting position by lifting buoys up to the surface. Repeat. Strengthens and tones triceps and biceps.

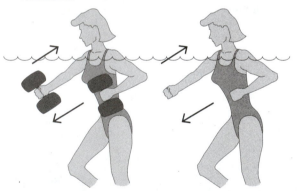

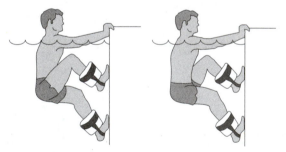

PUNCHES

With body leaning forward, punch arms downward and away from chest. NOTE: This exercise can be done with or without hand buoys. Strengthens and tones biceps, triceps, pectorals, and deltoids.

WALL STRIDES

Grip the wall with both hands, keeping arms shoulder distance apart. Place one foot at hip level on the wall. Place the other foot on the wall with leg fully extended. Push legs away from the wall, alternating foot placement. Strengthens and tones thighs and buttocks.

TIP: Push away from the wall with the balls of your feet. Stabilize your lower back by holding abdominals tight.

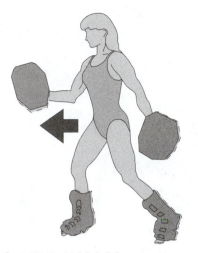

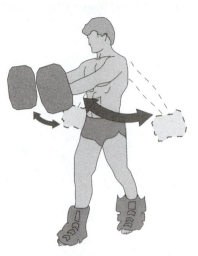

POWER WALK

With your HYDRO-BOOTS securely fastened and your HYDRO-BELLS in hand, POWER WALK around the shallow end of the pool for two minutes. This is a great warmup exercise.

TIP: Waist-deep water is best.

FRONT RAISES – PRESSDOWNS

With the water bells at your sides, vigorously raise them forward with straight arms and press downward to your sides. Exercises your lats (upper back) and front shoulders.

TIP: Begin upward movement from slightly behind you.

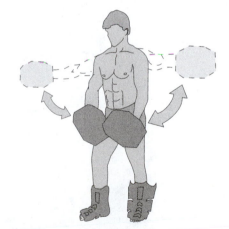

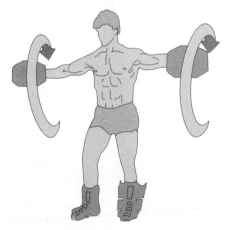

LATERAL RAISES – PRESSDOWNS

Raise and lower your HYDRO-BELLS sideward and back down vigorously. Exercises your shoulder and back muscles.

TIP: Begin with bells in front or in back of you.

ARM CIRCLES

With arms extended to the side, vigorously make big, sweeping circles downward for thirty seconds, and then reverse the motion for another thirty seconds. Exercises the muscles of the shoulder girdle.

TIP: May be done more rapidly with smaller arm circles. Vary hand position (palm up/palm down).

Hydro-Tone Exercises (continued)

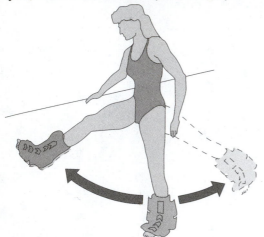

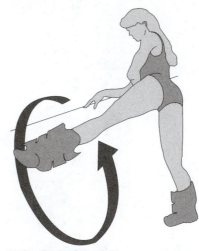

LEG KICKS

Holding onto the side of the pool, kick your leg forward and backward vigorously for 40-45 seconds. Repeat this exercise with your other leg. Exercises your hip and thigh muscles.
TIP: Keep leg straight and kick high.

LEG CIRCLES

Holding onto the side of the pool, vigorously make a big circle with your leg. Repeat this exercise with the opposite leg. Exercises all of your hip and thigh muscles.
TIP: Keep foot sidewards during kick – not toes first.

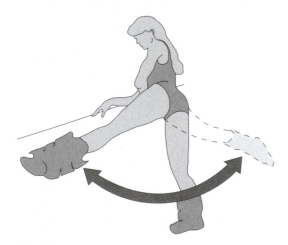

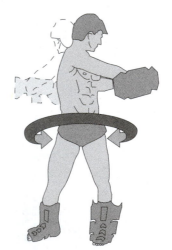

HIP SHAPER

With both hands on the pool's edge, stand with feet apart shoulder width. Vigorously raise one leg sidewards toward the surface of the water, and then draw it back downward, passing behind the stationary leg. Exercises the buttocks and hip flexor.
TIP: Keep toes pointed and knee up.

WAIST TRIMMER CIRCLES

Holding your HYDRO-BELLS slightly in front of you, vigorously circle left and right for 15-20 seconds. Exercises your sides and abdomen.
TIP: Use wide stance for stability.

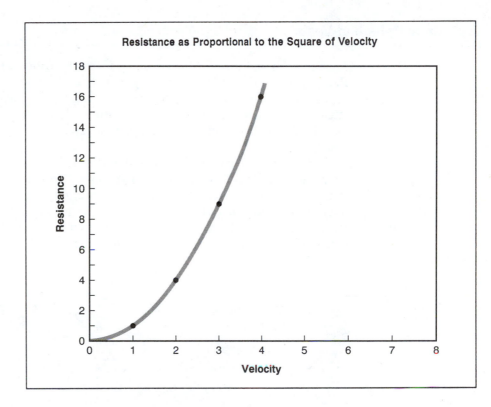

Aqua Paddles

Aqua paddles can be used to enhance your workout either muscularly or aerobically, or both, depending on how they are used. Aqua paddles are a type of water-resistive equipment that provides variable resistance. The resistance of the paddles may be increased or decreased with the simple movement of dials that are found at both ends of the paddles. With a simple flick of the wrist, muscles may be isolated and exercised.

Aqua Paddle Program Tips

When creating an aqua paddle workout on your own, be sure to select exercises that work all your opposing muscles to ensure the equal development of all of your muscles. Also, be careful not to overload your muscles too quickly. Use the progressive overload principle by increasing the resistance of the dial on the paddles gradually. Save all of your deltoid exercises for last, in order not to overtrain them—the deltoids act as muscle stabilizers and assistors most of the time when you are performing other exercises. A fun training idea that will help you avoid muscle overload is to play "Beat the Clock." This is done by timing how many repetitions, with perfect form, you can perform within a specific time period. Each day, try to keep the time the same but increase your repetitions by one or two. You will be able to see an improvement in your muscular endurance and strength over time.

Buoyancy Belts and Vests

Aquatic belts and vests under various trademarks (AquaJogger, Hydro-Tone Belt, Hydro-Fit Belt, Sprint Buoyancy Belt, The Wet Vest, Wet Belt, Stingray, etc.) are available to assist your buoyancy and allow you to experience zero (no) impact, deep-water workouts. Deep-water workouts allow you variety in aerobic as well as muscular conditioning. Chapter 11 describes deep-water workouts in detail.

Large-sized water wings, similar to those used by young children for buoyancy assistance, can be placed on your ankles and/or upper arms to allow you to participate in deep-water workouts while utilizing very inexpensive equipment. These water wings can be purchased in an aquatic supply store or in your local children's toy store. Nonswimmers are not advised to use this form of equipment in deep-water workouts, because they could be placed in danger if the water wings deflated.

Various buoyancy belts are available to provide non-impact, deep-water workouts.

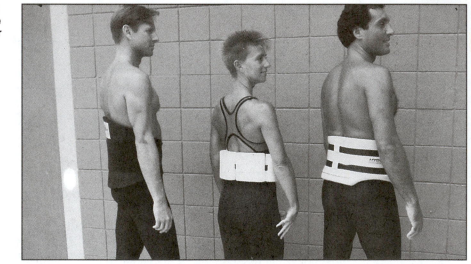

Dyna Bands

Dyna bands, also known as thera bands, are now produced by several companies under various names. The stretch bands are approximately four to six inches wide and come color coded, representing various tensile strengths. Strips are cut in lengths appropriate to the types of exercise the participant will execute.

Dyna bands can be used by standing on the center of a long strip and pulling up to work the biceps. Repeat ten times.

Pull back on the band and press up and resist the return. Repeat ten times.

Hold the band at chest level, pull out, and resist the return. Repeat ten times.

Tie and knot the end of the band, and place the band around your thighs. Balance on one leg and hold on to the wall for support. Lift your leg to the side

Dyna band, pull up

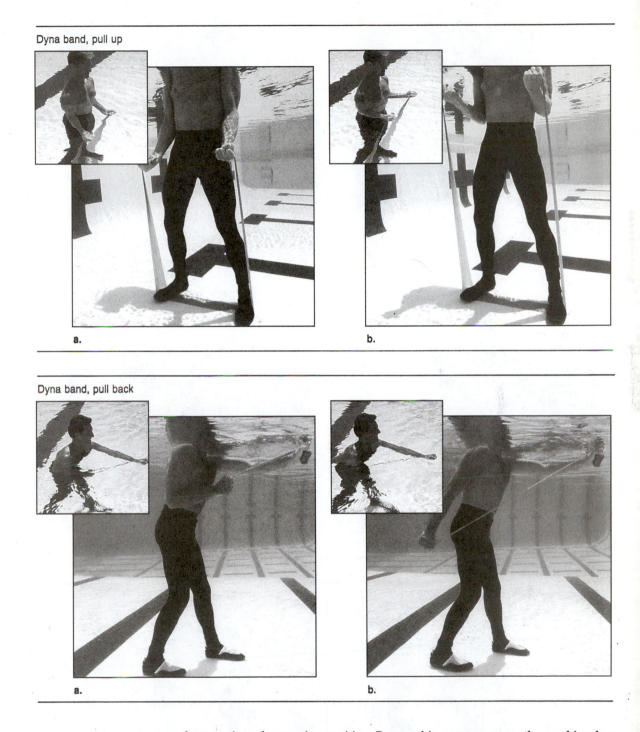

a.

b.

Dyna band, pull back

a.

b.

and return it to the starting position. Repeat this movement on the working leg 20 times, then change legs and begin again.

Use a band that has been tied together. Stand on one part of the circle with one foot and place the instep of the other foot on the curve of the band. Keep both knees together throughout the movement. Lift the working foot up toward the buttocks, and then slowly lower it. Repeat 20 times on each leg.

Dyna band, pull out

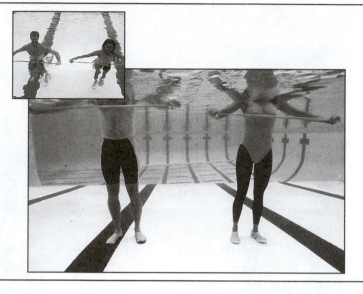

Dyna band, thighs

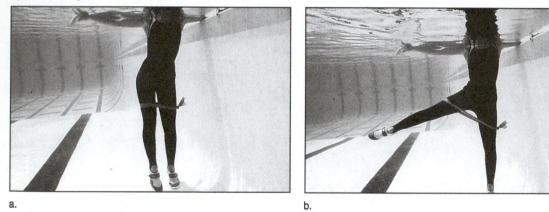

a.   b.

Dyna band, hamstring

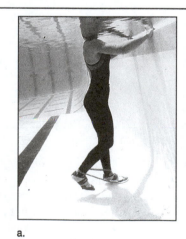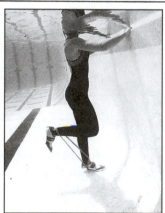

a.   b.

Pull Buoys

Pull buoys are intended to be used between the upper thighs to offer buoyancy to the legs when you are swimming only with your arms in order to perfect your arm strokes. However, they can also be adapted for use in a variety of aquatic strengthening exercises for the upper and lower body. When held by the straps or placed under the armpit, pull buoys will support your body in a manner similar to the dumbbell-type flotation devices. Some participants need to use two pull buoys in each hand to obtain the same flotation benefits as one dumbbell. Pull buoys can be substituted in all of the exercises previously described that use dumbbell flotation devices. Additionally, there are several lower-body exercises in which pull buoys can be used. Similar exercises, which used cuffs on the ankles, were described in the Hydro-Fit Equipment section.

Hamstring Exercises

Place the strap of the pull buoy over the instep of your foot to add resistance to your movements. Stand, with your body in good alignment and your abdominal muscles pulled in, facing the side wall of the pool, with your hands on the wall for support. Keeping your legs parallel and your knees close together, bend at the knee and slowly lift your right foot up toward the buttocks. Then slowly return the right foot to the start position. Repeat 20 times. Change the buoy to the other foot and perform the exercise 20 times. Repeat this exercise on both sides.

Leg Lift Back

With the pull buoy on your instep, execute the leg lift back exercises described in Chapter 7.

Pull buoy, hamstring

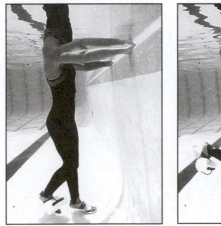
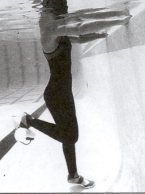

a.   b.

Pull buoy, leg lift back

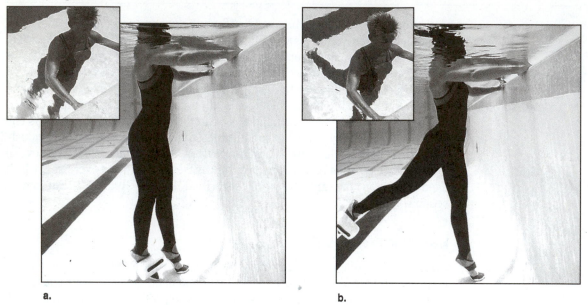

a.   b.

Crossover Figure Eights

See the description in Chapter 7. Perform this exercise in its entirety with the pull buoy on the instep of one foot. Repeat on the other foot.

Developpé

Stand in good alignment, with your side to the side wall of the pool. Hold onto the wall for support. With the pull buoy placed on the instep of the foot which is away from the wall, slightly rotate your legs out at the thighs so that the heels almost touch and the toes face each diagonal. (This is first position in ballet.) Keeping the leg turned out from the thigh, begin gradually lifting the foot up so that the toes pass the supporting knee. When the working leg reaches a 90° angle, extend the foot forward (to a straight leg position) and then pull a straight leg down and backward through the water to return to the starting position. Repeat 10 times. Keeping the working leg turned out so that the toes face a diagonal, repeat the exercise on the diagonal 10 times. Finally, repeat to the back.

Caution

When lifting to the back, you are just to go as high as you can—it is impossible to get to a 90° angle to the back. Be sure to keep your back straight, stomach pulled in, and your body in good alignment throughout the developpé.

Pull buoy, developpé

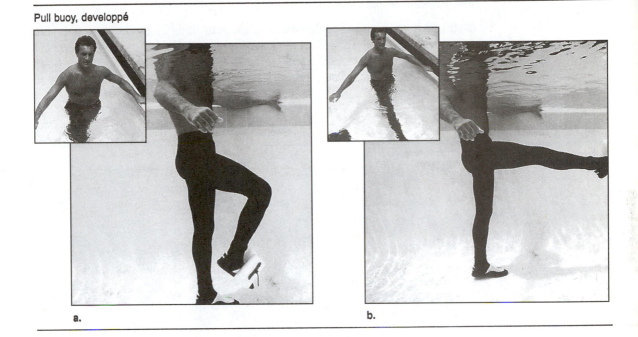

a.   b.

Swings Side to Side

Standing in good alignment, hold one arm and buoy straight out to the right side of the body, directly under the water's surface, with the other arm bent across the chest. Swing your hands and arms from one side of the body to the other in a smooth, relaxed manner.

Pull buoy, swing side to side

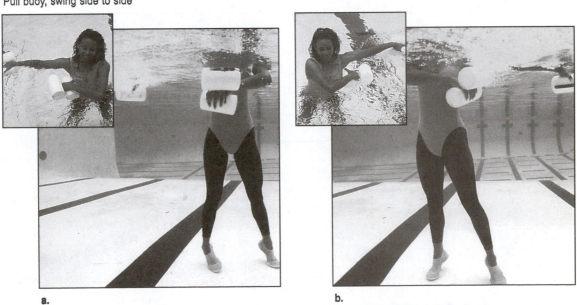

a.   b.

Pec Press in Front

Stand with your legs shoulder-width apart, your body in good alignment, your knees soft, and your abdominal muscles contracted. Hold the buoys out to each side. Press the buoys under the water and toward the midline of the body. Pressing through the water, return to the starting position. Repeat the movements 20 times.

Pull buoy, pec press in front

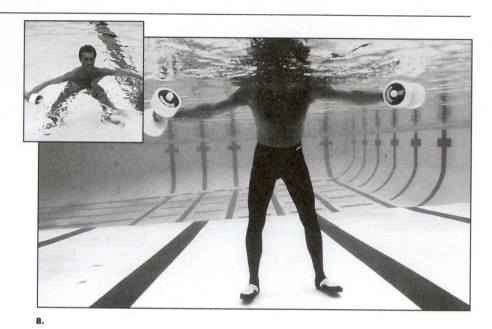

a.

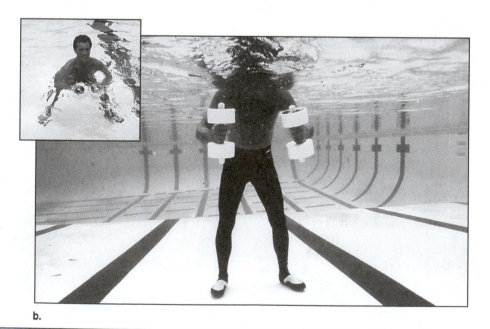

b.

Rhomboid Press Behind

Begin in the same position described for the pec press in front. Press the buoys through the water behind your body. Press through the water to return to the starting position. Repeat the movements 20 times.

Pull buoy, rhomboid press behind

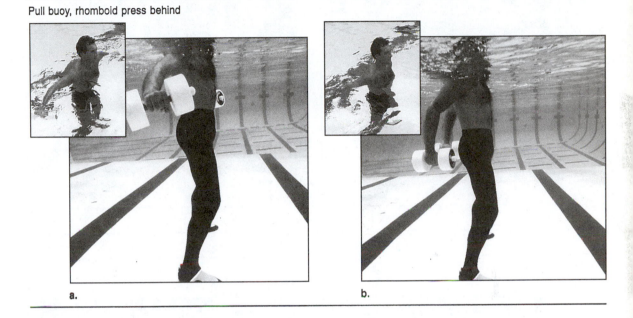

a.   b.

Other Pull Buoy Options

The following exercises, which were described in Chapter 7, can be performed holding the pull buoys or dumbbells to add resistance to the movement: roller, biceps and triceps press, arm flies, breast stroke—arms, and all other pectoral presses.

Kickboard

Press Down

Stand in waist- to shoulder-deep water in good alignment. Hold a kickboard in front of your body, on and parallel to the surface of the water. Place your palms on top of the board. Using both hands equally, press the kickboard down, under the water. Next, change your grip so that your palms are under the board, facing the surface of the water. Pull the board up through the water, keeping it parallel to the surface throughout the movement. Repeat 20 times.

Variation: Stand in shoulder-deep water, holding the kickboard perpendicular to the water's surface with your hands on each side of the board. Begin with the kickboard parallel to and close to your chest. Push and press the board through the water until your arms are extended. Pull the board back through the water to return to the starting position. Repeat 20 times.

These exercises strengthen the chest area (pectoralis major and minor) as well as the biceps and triceps.

Kickboard, press down

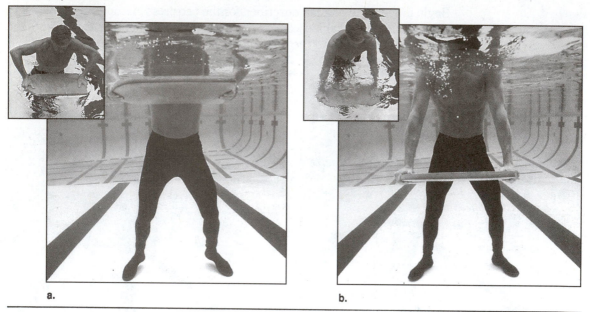

a.   b.

Kickboard, press out

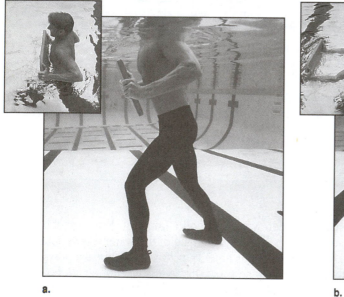
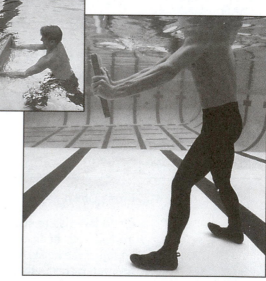

a.   b.

Twist While Holding Board

Stand in a balanced, well-grounded position. Hold the board perpendicular to the water, lengthwise. While holding the board in front of your body and moving only the upper body, twist all the way to the left and then to the right. Perform in a smooth, rhythmical manner 10 times.

This exercise works the abdominal area, back, and shoulder girdle.

Twist while holding board

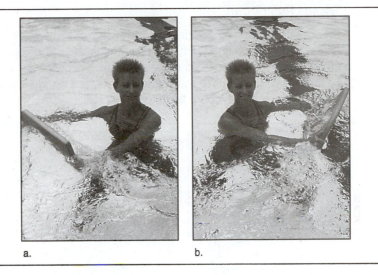

a.   b.

Run With Board

Stand in waist- to armpit-level water and place the board in front of you, width-wise, on the surface of the water. Put one hand on each side of the board. Slightly tilt the top of the board in the water on a diagonal away from you to add resistance, and jog forward through the water holding the board in this manner. Jog through the shallow end of the pool completing one to four lengths or widths of the pool. Add a length or a width of jogging in this manner each week.

This will work your legs and cardiovascular respiratory system harder than if you were jogging through the water without added resistance.

Run with board

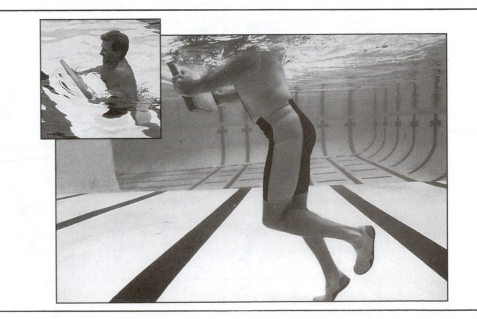

Triceps Push Down

Stand with your feet shoulder-width apart and the body in good alignment. Place the board behind your back, parallel to the water's surface. Keeping your elbows pointing back, hold the board with one hand on each side. Press the board down through the water and pull it back up. Repeat this exercise 15-25 times. This exercise works the triceps muscles.

Kickboard, triceps push down

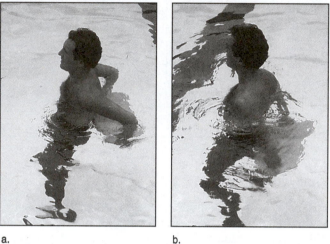

a.   b.

Rubber Ball

Pendulum

Stand with your feet shoulder-width apart. Hold the ball in both hands to the right diagonal of your body. In a smooth manner, press the ball under the water and make a half-circle motion to the left until you end up with the ball on the left diagonal to the surface of the water. Repeat, moving in the other direction. Repeat the entire exercise 10 times.

This exercise works the arms, erector muscles, and rhomboids.

Rubber ball, pendulum

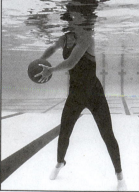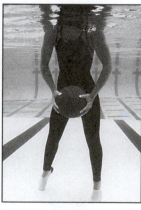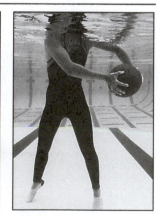

a.   b.   c.

Full Circles

Stand with your legs shoulder-width apart in proper body alignment. Hold the ball in both hands with arms extended over the head. Make a full circle with the ball beginning in the air and then moving through the water, as in the pendulum movement described above. Execute five circles in each direction.

Caution

Move very slowly to avoid placing stress on your shoulder joints, since you are transferring from air resistance to water resistance.

Rubber ball, full circles

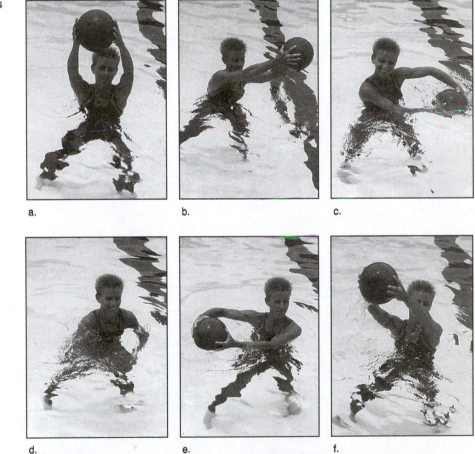

a.   b.   c.

d.   e.   f.

Triceps Extender

Stand with your feet shoulder-width apart and your body in good alignment. Hold the ball with both hands overhead. Slowly lower the ball to a position with the elbows toward the sky and the ball facing the bottom of the pool, behind your head. Then return to the starting position. Repeat 10 times. This exercise works the triceps muscles.

Rubber ball, triceps extender

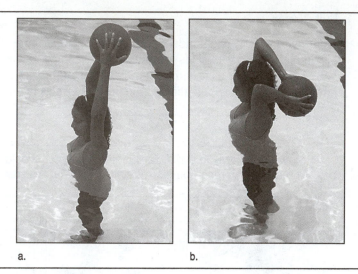

a.   b.

Paddle-Pull

Begin in waist-deep water. Place the ball between your knees and calves, and squeeze them close around the ball. Assume a sitting-type position in the water, with your torso upright. Keeping the abdominal muscles tight throughout the movement, use your arms to pull yourself across the pool with breast-stroke or "dog paddle" arm movements. Paddle-pull yourself several lengths or widths of the pool. This exercise works your adductor muscles, your arms, and your abdominals.

Rubber ball, paddle-pull

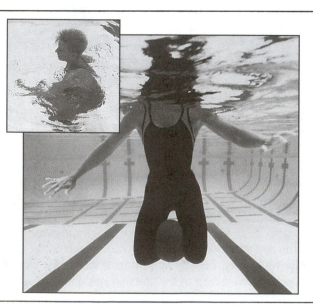

Webbed Gloves

Webbed gloves can be worn throughout your workout in order to increase the resistance to your arm movements.

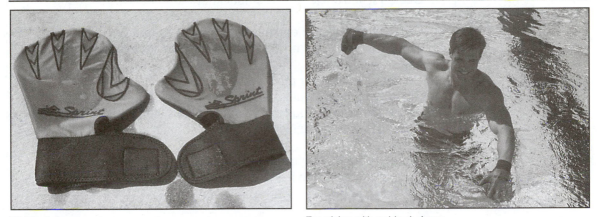

Webbed gloves   Exercising with webbed gloves

Purchasing Equipment

Before you purchase equipment, it is wise to test it out. See if your instructor knows of a source where you can try out equipment before you buy it. Another place to inquire about equipment rental is your local aquatic supply vendor, who may be able to lend or rent you equipment before you purchase it. Find out what your instructor knows about the various types of equipment on the market and the pros and cons of each type. Your instructor knows you and can probably offer advice that will guide you toward the equipment best suited to help you meet your personal fitness goals.

Checklist: Aqua Aerobics Equipment

1. Decide if you'd like to utilize equipment to enhance your aqua aerobics workout.
2. Select the type(s) of equipment you'd like to use (your instructor can give you advice on what equipment will be best suited to your goals and needs).
3. Contact a vendor for purchasing information.
4. Check your local aquatic supply store to see if they sell or can obtain the type of equipment you are interested in using, and see if you can test the equipment before committing yourself to a purchase.
5. Once you have purchased the equipment, carefully read the instructions before trying it out in your pool.

Summary

1. The equipment available for aqua aerobics can be used to enhance and provide variety to your class workout.
2. A variety of equipment is available for purchase, including:

   - Hydro-Fit.
   - Hydro-Tone.
   - Aqua paddles.
   - Buoyancy belts and vests.
   - Dyna Bands.
   - Dumbbell-type flotation/resistance equipment or pull buoys.
   - Webbed gloves.
   - Kickboards.
   - Rubber balls.

3. Ask your instructor for advice on equipment before you purchase it.
4. The types of equipment available can assist you with zero (no) impact deep-water workouts and provide additional resistance to increase your overall conditioning level.
5. Check with your local aquatic supply vendor to see if they sell equipment specialized for aquatic aerobic exercise and if you can test it out before making a purchase.

CHAPTER 11

Deep-Water Workouts

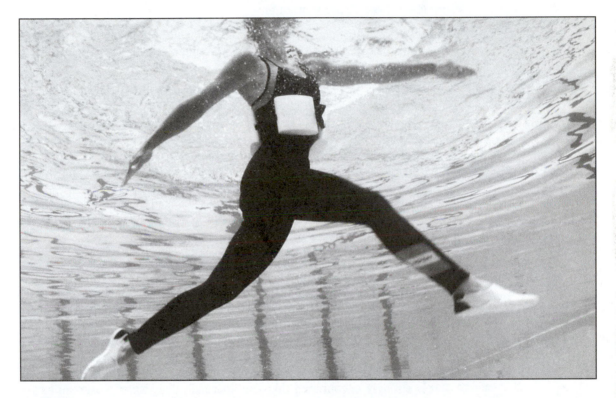

Outline

Introduction—What Are Deep-Water Workouts?

Deep-water workouts are unique aquatic exercise techniques that are appropriate for participants at any level of fitness. With the aid of a specialized flotation vest or belt, participants are suspended in the water, preferably without their feet touching the pool bottom. Movements will involve use of the hands, arms, torso, abdomen, legs, and feet, thus creating a total body workout.

Benefits of Deep-Water Workouts

Deep-water workouts complement all components of water exercise, with additional rewards as well. The features that distinguish this technique from traditional water exercise programs are:

1. The body is suspended in the water—thus *zero impact* is placed on the musculoskeletal system.
2. A specialized vest or belt is used to assist in keeping the head above water.
3. The weight of the water compresses the entire ribcage and increases the pressure on the lungs, thereby causing the respiratory muscles to work harder. Therefore, exercising in this submerged (from the neck down) state increases the effectiveness of the exercise on the lungs.
4. Since the body is submerged to the neck the water provides constant resistance in every direction, causing muscles to work concentrically and thereby eliminating or reducing muscle soreness.

Concepts and Properties of Deep-Water Exercising

The training effects of deep-water workouts are based on the principles of hydrodynamic resistance (commonly referred to as hydrotherapy in the medical profession) instead of gravitational resistance, as used in weight training. Concepts similar to those used in deep-water exercising are applied in the vigorous training that United States astronauts undergo in a neutral buoyancy tank—water is the medium used to create a feeling of weightlessness.

It is strongly encouraged that you approach deep-water workouts as you would a new sport. You need to train your body to execute upper- and lower-body movements while maintaining safe and effective body alignment in the deep water.

Isodynamics

Movements executed in deep-water workouts are performed at a constant speed or with spurts of faster movements and use the resistance of the water or additional resistance equipment. Constant speed movement has been termed *isodynamics* by deep-water running expert J. Glenn McWaters. Muscles receive equal amounts of tension from the pressure of the water on the body. The more quickly you move, the more resistance you will experience. In a land-based program, isokinetic movements or "same speed" muscle contractions would be similar. Mr. McWaters has replaced kinetic with dynamic because that is exactly the way the water movements will feel to your muscles! In his book *Sports Psychology*, Edward Fox states: "From a theoretical viewpoint, isokinetic contractions (isodynamic in the water) and thus isokinetic training programs appear to be best suited for improving athletic performance."

Buoyancy

Buoyancy can be defined as the ability or tendency to be suspended in liquid or air. The natural buoyancy of the exerciser, combined with the vest or belt utilized in deep-water workouts, will completely support the body in the water while keeping the head comfortably above the water. Make sure that your flotation belt is fastened securely around your midsection and keeps your head above the water. The belt or vest should fit snugly, but not so tightly that it constricts breathing. The belt should not slide up your back or into your ribs. There are several types of vests or belts on the market today. Try them out and use the type that works best for you. (Appendix F lists the various sources from which to purchase equipment.)

When you are wearing a buoyancy vest/belt, your feet will not touch the bottom of the pool; this creates the ultimate exercise environment with *zero impact*. In addition, your body is completely surrounded and buoyed by water, thus virtually eliminating the risk of injury.

The Importance of Relaxing

It is essential for you to be comfortable and relaxed in your pool environment so that you will reap the full benefits of deep-water workouts. Please remember that you are in control when exercising. You must work at your own pace and your own level of intensity. There is no place in an exercise program for exhaustion or competition with a neighbor!

Muscles that are tense from fear or chilled from cold water do not perform well. To help you relax, you need to be aware of the following conditions prior to beginning your deep-water experience: water depth, space requirements, and progression of training.

Water Depth. It is best to exercise in a depth of water that will completely cushion your body. Your height will determine the specific depth necessary for you. For most people, a depth of seven feet and deeper is appropriate. If you are fearful of not being able to place your feet on the bottom, begin at a depth where you can touch the bottom of the pool with your toes. As you gain confidence in yourself, are more comfortable in the vest or belt, and feel like you are completely in control of your body, then you can move into deeper water.

Space Requirements. It is important for you to be able to move about freely in the water and not feel confined by another person sharing your space. If the deep-water area of your pool is very small, you can purchase a tether that attaches from the vest or belt to a ladder of the pool and allows you freedom of movement without constantly having to turn around in a restricted area.

Principles of Deep-Water Exercise Training

Body Alignment

The first technique that you must acquire is that of effective and safe "water posture," or deep-water body alignment. The vest or belt will suspend your body upright in the water and keep your head comfortably above water. To obtain proper alignment, concentrate on feeling as if you are being pulled by the top of your head to stretch the length of your spine. Simultaneously, contract the abdominals and tilt the pelvis down and slightly forward. Your arms should be relaxed comfortably at your sides. To visualize yourself from the side in proper alignment, imagine a plumbline hanging from your mastoid process (behind the ear) and going through your shoulder, hip, and ankle.

Duration, Frequency, and Intensity of Activity

The principles of duration, frequency, and intensity of activity are the same for shallow- and deep-water aquatic exercise activities and have been explained in detail in Chapter 2. When adapting to the deep-water environment, you should begin working at a level of short duration and low intensity and progress gradually. Once you have comfortably accomplished continuous movement in the deep water for 20 minutes or longer, you should begin increasing the intensity of your workout. Begin with intervals or bursts of energy, as opposed to attempting to maintain the same pace throughout the entire workout. Before you know it, your bursts of energy will last longer and the rests in between will be shorter. Listen to your body and respond accordingly. The important thing is to maintain continuous movement.

Determining Target Heart Rate for Deep-Water Workouts

Target heart rate was described in Chapter 2 as the minimum rate at which your heart should be beating in order to achieve a safe and optimally effective level for aerobic improvement. The most popular formula utilized for land-based aerobic activity and shallow-water workouts is the Karvonen formula (described in Chapter 2). However, when you exercise in deep water at the same exertion level as in shallow water or on land, your heart rate is *lower*. According to Glenn McWaters, in his book *Deep Water Exercise for Health and Fitness*, "The decreased gravitational pull is believed to be the main factor in the reduced heart rate. Another factor is that your extremities are subjected to more pressure in the water than they are in the air. This increased pressure forces the blood from the extremities back to the heart at a faster rate; thus, more blood is available to be pumped by the heart. Reduced gravitational pull on the heart and increased rate of return of blood to the heart mean that the heart doesn't have to work as hard to produce an efficient cardiovascular workout."

During submaximal exercise, the heart rate is about 10 to 15 beats per minute less; at maximal level (for trained athletes in a specific sports program) the heart rate is about 20 beats less per minute. The Karvonen formula has thus been modified to address these specifications for deep-water exercisers—instead of using 220 beats per minute as the maximum heart rate, begin your calculations based on 205 beats per minute as the maximum rate.

Note

Resting heart rate is not used in the modification of the Karvonen formula listed on the following page.

For example: 205
                – 40   (Put in your own age)
                ────
                 165   (predicted maximum heart rate)
                x .7   (70% of predicted heart rate)
                ────
                 115   (lower end of training zone)

                 205
                – 40   (age)
                ────
                 165   (predicted maximum heart rate)
                x .85   (85% of predicted heart rate)
                ────
                 140   (upper end of training zone)

Thus, for a 40-year-old, the training heart rate zone is 115 to 140 beats per minute to maintain a 70 to 85 percent level of intensity for cardiovascular conditioning.

Rate of Perceived Exertion Adapted for Deep-Water Exercise

Due to the unique characteristics of a deep-water exercise program, Glenn McWaters has revised the Borg scale of perceived exertion (see Chapter 2) to better fit the activity.

Borg/McWaters Modified Ratings of Perceived Exertion

0	Nothing at all
1	Very, very weak
2	Very weak
3	Weak
4	Somewhat weak
5	Moderate
6	Somewhat hard
7	Hard
8	Very hard
9	Very, very hard
10	Maximal (all-out effort)

The Deep-Water Workout Format

The format of a deep-water workout is very similar to that of a shallow-water exercise program, consisting of the following phases:

Warm-up phase	5 to 10 minutes
Cardiovascular conditioning phase	20 to 45 minutes
Muscular strength and endurance phase	10 minutes
Stretching/wall-work phase	10 minutes

The objectives of the four phases of a deep-water workout are the same as they are for shallow-water workouts. The cardiovascular conditioning and muscular strength/endurance phases can be combined. Be sure to end your workout with the stretching/wall-work phase. Remember, exhaustion has no place in your exercise program!

Putting It All Together

This section will describe and illustrate a number of deep-water movements that have been designed to concentrate on various muscle groups. These are, of course, only a few of the virtually endless combinations of exercises you could perform during a deep-water workout.

The following guidelines should be adhered to when performing any of the movements shown on the following pages.

1. Safe and effective body alignment must be attained before you perform any movements other than walking or running in your vest or belt. To accomplish this, hold your abdominal muscles in, tuck your buttocks down and slightly under, and press your shoulders down. Feel tall and keep your chest open. Try not to slouch. Keep your toes in line with your knees.
2. Always keep your arms where you can see them; do not allow them to go behind your shoulders. In a deep-water workout, pulled-back arms cannot only put stress on your shoulders but can also cause your back to arch and create a stress on the mid to lower back.
3. Keep your hips in line with your shoulders. If you feel like you are falling forward, you must hold your abdominals in and tuck your hips under your shoulders.
4. Contract your abdominal muscles throughout your workout. This is the one single contraction that will flatten your stomach and strengthen not only the abdominals, but your lower back as well.
5. When kicking in the water, you need not bend the knee beyond a 90° angle. If you have any knee problems or are rehabilitating your knee(s), restrict your range of motion. Go by how it feels. It's okay to feel a mild discomfort, but not sharp pain.
6. Flexion and extension of the hands and feet are encouraged after the warm-up to increase the resistance of the water; however, if these movements cause discomfort or cramping (especially in the feet) do not continue.
7. Take care not to let your head fall back into your shoulders and apply pressure on the cervical vertebrae. This could cause you to draw your shoulders up to support your head and lead to a stiff, tight upper neck and back. Keep your chin parallel to the water. If you are swallowing water when you try to breathe, then you need a different flotation device or additional flotation equipment.
8. Work at your own pace and your own level of intensity. Don't rush the movements. If you want to move fast, shorten your range of motion. Likewise, if you want to slow down, increase your range of motion. Depending on your current fitness level and program goals, you do not always have to go fast to elevate the heart rate.
9. Listen to your body *always*. If it's telling you to slow down, then respond accordingly.

10. If you are an athlete with a desire to design a sport-specific program to enhance your performance, simply take your land workout into the water and perform it in basically the same manner. Deep-water workouts have been utilized to enhance performance in activities including running, football, basketball, baseball, tennis, gymnastics, and dancing, just to name a few. More and more athletic trainers are integrating water workouts into their training programs to enhance an athlete's performance or for rehabilitation. Deep-water exercise programs have demonstrated physical as well as mental benefits not only to healthy athletes but injured athletes as well—the ability to maintain a training program helps the competitive athlete maintain a positive mental attitude while rehabilitating.

Deep-Water Walking

The body is in the water in a vertical position. Maintain proper body alignment while walking during your deep-water workout. Progress slowly through the water as you would on dry land. Relax your arms along the sides of your body, swinging alternate arms forward and backward through the water. Move at your own pace within your range of motion.

If you want to increase the intensity of your walking, try one of the following:

- Shorten your range of motion and increase the speed of your walking movement.
- Flex your hands at the wrist and press down with the palms of your hands while flexing your feet at the ankles.
- Use aquatic resistance equipment (webbed gloves, paddles, dumbbells, etc.)

> *Caution*
>
> Master deep-water walking before progressing to deep-water running.

Deep-Water Running

Lean forward slightly in the water, as if you were running outdoors. Progress slowly through the water, using the exact same motion as you would on land. Keep your arms beside your body with elbows bent at a 90° angle, propelling them forward and backward.

If you want to increase the resistance on your upper body, cup your hands or add webbed gloves. If you need to decrease the resistance on your upper body, keep your hands open and do not wear gloves.

The overall intensity of your running can be increased by:

- Increasing your pace.
- Running intervals.
- Using aquatic resistance equipment.

Be careful not to lean too far forward when you run as you will decrease the resistance, thus decreasing the intensity of your overall workout.

Deep-water running

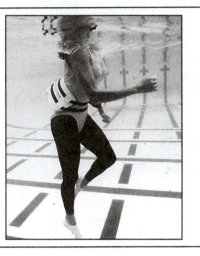

Overstriding Exercise (A Variation of Running)

Assume a natural running position. Lift one knee high, then reach out with your foreleg as far as it will go, getting full extension. Simultaneously extend the other leg toward the rear as far as it will go. Alternate your legs as if running on land. Keep your toes and knees straight ahead. The elbows are bent at a 90° angle throughout the overstriding exercise. On the backward motion, your arms move straight back with the tricep barely touching the surface of the water. On the forward arm motion, the fist will come close to the surface of the water.

Upper-Body Movements

These exercises include hands, fingers, wrists, forearms, biceps, triceps, shoulders, latissimus dorsi, deltoids, trapezius, and pectoralis.

Hands, fingers, and wrists:

1. Keep hands open, fingers stretched apart.
2. Close hands with the fingers together in a loose fist.
3. Cup hands.

Deep-water overstriding

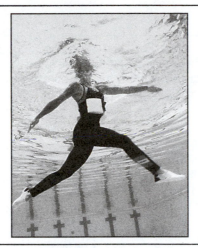

4. Open and close fingers during execution of arm movements.
5. Flex and extend wrists.
6. Make wrist circles.

Forearms, biceps, and triceps:

1. Alternately press, punch, or reach the arms to the front of the body.
2. Simultaneously press, punch, or reach the arms to the front of the body.
3. Simultaneously press, punch, or reach the arms out to the side of the body.
4. Alternately press, punch, or reach the arms down toward the pool bottom.
5. Simultaneously press, punch, or reach the arms down toward the pool bottom.
6. Combine movements of the press, punch, or reach forward on a 1–2 count and then out to the sides on a 3–4 count.
7. Alternately press, punch, or reach one arm to the front and the other to the side on a 1–2 count and then switch arms on a 3–4 count.

Deep-water arm
punching

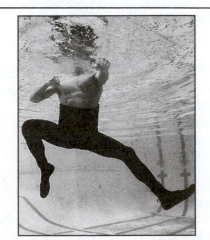

Caution

If utilizing movements 1, 2, 3, 6, and 7 in the warm-up phase, keep the arms to the front of the body with the elbows in front of the shoulders; once the muscles are warmed up, the elbows can slide back beyond the shoulder joint.

---

8. Alternate bicep curls.
9. Simultaneous bicep curls.
10. Alternate tricep press.
11. Simultaneous tricep press.
12. Tricep extensions to the side.

Deep-water bicep curl

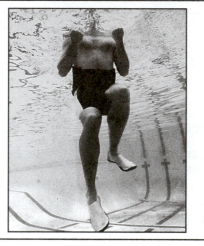

Note

In Exercises 8 through 12 the elbow is the lever and the upper arm is kept steady while the movement is executed with the forearm. Resistance equipment can be utilized to vary the intensity.

Shoulders, Latissimus dorsi, deltoids, trapezius, and pectoralis:

1. Shoulder rolls—Roll shoulders forward and in reverse (shoulders can be rolled simultaneously or alternately).
2. Funky chicken—Position elbows out and hands to the center of your body, palms down. Keeping the hands steady, flap the elbows like wings while pressing up and down.
3. Fanning your body—With the palms of your hands toward your chest (elbows out to the side), keep your upper arms steady while your forearms open and close simultaneously or alternately.
4. Press aways—Press hands forward from the chest; variations can be created by manipulating the hands.

5. Arm circles—Arms can circle in both directions, varying the intensity by the size and pace of the circles.
6. Hand clapping—Clap hands together slowly within a large range of motion or increase the pace and clap quickly.
7. Crazy misclaps—Make a clapping motion as one arm/hand crosses over the other; alternate arm on top. Variation: turn palms of hands outward, with the thumbs down.

Caution

In the execution of exercises 6 and 7, the arms can be extended or the elbows can be flexed. Do not keep the arms stiff—it is essential that you do not feel any strain or pain in the shoulders or upper back.

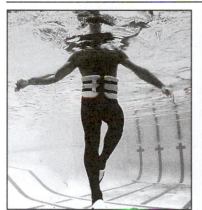 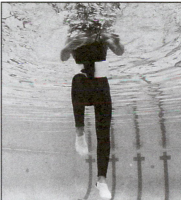 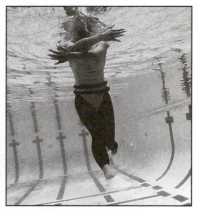

Deep-water arm circles   Deep-water hand clapping   Deep-water crazy misclaps

Midsection

These exercises include lower back, abdominals, and obliques.

1. Contract abdominals throughout the exercises. This will not only strengthen and flatten your tummy but also nurture a stronger, healthier lower back.
2. Swivel hips—With both arms, reach across the center of your body toward the opposite hip; gently swivel or rotate that hip opposite to the direction you are reaching. Allow your body to be relaxed and do not perform this movement quickly. Do not twist or use the lower back as a pivot point.
3. Crossovers—Press, punch, or reach your arms out in front, across the center of your body toward the opposite foot or knee. Keep the legs in line with the hips.

Legwork

These exercises include feet, ankles, knees, adductors/abductors, hamstrings, quadriceps, calves, buttocks, and hip flexors.

Deep-water hip swivel

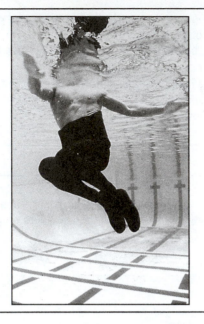

Feet and ankles:

1. Keep feet relaxed, as if large flippers are on your feet.
2. Flex or extend at the ankles.
3. Point or curl toes.
4. Make ankle circles.

Knees, hamstrings, quadriceps, hip flexor, buttocks, and calves:

1. Kicking—When executing a movement such as a kick from the knee, you do not want to bend the knee in excess of 90° (the angle at back of the knee). If you feel any pain or discomfort, immediately decrease the intensity of the movement or discontinue altogether.
2. Skipping—Alternate lifting the legs from the hips with knees slightly flexed; the height of the leg lift is up to you, but always maintain good body alignment. Keep your legs in line with your hips.
3. Marching—Flex knees at a 90° angle; pressing down with the heels of your feet (feet are flexed), alternate lifting and pressing your legs up and down.
4. Cowboy kicks—Kick your legs out (simultaneously or alternately) at a 60° angle to your body. The height of your leg kicks is up to you, but the highest you should go is level with the hips.
5. Leg extensions—With both legs together, out in front of the body, flex knees no more than 90° and then extend legs back out to their starting position in front of your body. Legs are extended and flexed simultaneously.
6. Cycling—Pedal your legs as if riding a bike. Variations: (1) cycle backwards; (2) cycle while lying on your side.

> ### *Caution*
>
> In exercises 4, 5, and 6, keep the legs in front of the body at hip level or below.

Deep-water leg
extension

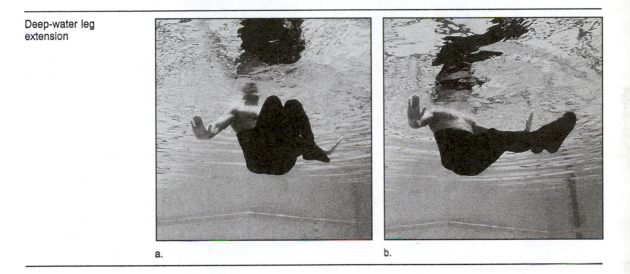

a.   b.

Deep-water cycling

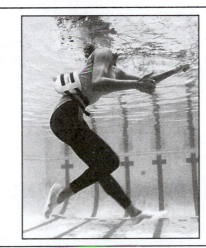

Adductor and abductor movements:

1. Jumping jacks—With feet relaxed or flexed and body position vertical in the water, simultaneously push legs apart and press them back together. Use arm movements that coordinate with the jacks.
2. Criss-cross—Feet are relaxed or flexed with the body vertical in the water. Push legs apart and alternate crossing one over the other when pressing the legs toward the center. (This is similar to the criss-cross described earlier in the text, with the use of dumbbells for flotation.)

Deep-water jumping jack

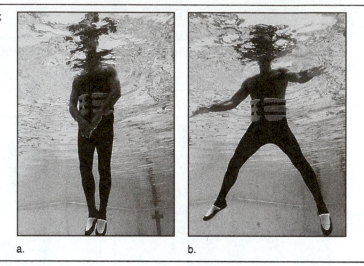

a.   b.

3. L-sit—Contract the abdominals and lift your legs in front of your body, no higher than your hips. Maintaining good body alignment, push the legs apart and then press them back together to the center. Feet can be relaxed or flexed. (This is similar to the criss-cross above, but executed in an L-sit position.)
4. Frog kicks—Put the bottoms of your feet together, with your knees turned out. Pull your heels in toward the groin and extend the legs back out to the center while keeping the knees turned out.
5. Thigh press—In a position similar to the one you would assume when sitting in a chair, keep the feet in line with the knees and simultaneously push your legs apart and then press them back together.

Combinations of Movements

You can combine any of the upper-body and lower-body movements by following these guidelines.

1. Perform movements within your range of motion.
2. Work at your own pace; intensity is increased with speed and/or range of motion. Slow down if you are feeling tired.
3. If it hurts, don't do it!
4. The number of repetitions you execute is entirely up to you.
5. Put sequences of movements together to work your entire body.

Examples of effective combinations include:

1. Bicep and tricep curls with marching.
2. Pressing, punching, or reaching forward with a kick.
3. Pressing, punching, or reaching to the side (and/or forward) with cowboy kicks.
4. Reaching and pulling the arms in front with a cycling motion.
5. Reaching or pressing arms out to the front with simultaneous leg extensions.

6. Pressing away with the arms and kicking with the legs.
7. Doing the funky chicken with the arms while marching with the legs. For a fun variation, vary the speed.
8. Reaching for the opposite foot with your hands/arms while lifting the leg up to the front from the buttocks.
9. Gently pressing to the sides or scooping with the arms while performing frog kicks.
10. Skipping with your legs while swinging your arms in opposition.

The Stretching Wall-Work Phase

The objectives of this phase of the workout are to:

1. Slow the movements down.
2. Execute a full range of motion.
3. Maintain a degree of warmth in the body to prevent chilling.

If you begin to shiver while you are stretching at the wall, you may wish to get out of the pool and stretch at the poolside.

Caution

While at the wall, maintain good body alignment and keep abdominals contracted throughout the exercises. You may remove your flotation device if you wish.

Muscles Worked in Stretching Wall-Work Movements

Muscles Worked	Movement
Hip flexor, gluteals, hamstrings, calves, and lower back	Running up the wall—Alternate legs up the wall as high as you can, allowing the hips to bob in the water. Be aware of body alignment throughout the exercise.
Hip flexor, gluteals, abdominals, hamstrings, and calves	Gently holding onto the side, with your body at a slight angle to the pool, keep your legs together and move from the hips. Moving slowly, alternate each leg forward until the toes "tap" the front wall, while gently pressing the other leg back as far as it can go without compromising body alignment. You do not want to feel anything in your back—if you do, decrease your pace and range of motion.

Muscles Worked	Movement
Hip flexor, gluteals, hamstrings, and abdominals	Hurdles: Maintain a 120° angle to the poolside. You may wish to place one hand down on the wall to assist in supporting your back. Keep your feet flexed. Alternate bringing the knees under the chest and pressing the legs back and forth through the water. If you feel any discomfort in your back, lower your legs immediately.
Abdominals, hip flexors, and gluteals	Abdominal curls—Maintain a 120° angle to the poolside. Facing the wall, lift your legs together up to the chest and then slowly extend them back down to their original position. This is a very controlled movement and should not be done quickly.
Quadriceps, hamstrings, and calves	Leg curls—The body is at a slight angle to the poolside, and the legs are together. Gently flex both feet and lift the heels up toward the gluteals. Release by extending the legs back down to their original position. Take care to keep the upper part of your legs steady while you do this exercise. Variation: alternate leg curls.
Mid-section, obliques, lower back, gluteals, and hips	Leg circles—Keep your back toward the wall while maintaining good body alignment. Your arms are comfortably holding on to the sides, and your legs are together out in front of the hips. Contract the abdominals and slowly push both legs around to the right as far as you can. Keeping the movement continuous, bring the legs under the body (vertically), slowly lift up to the left, and complete the circle back to the center. After several repetitions, repeat in the opposite direction.
Inner/outer thighs, calves, hamstrings, upper/lower back, and shoulders	Straddle stretch—Facing the wall, straddle your legs on the wall of the pool, keeping the legs hip-height.

Muscles Worked	Movement
	The toes should be turned comfortably outward in line with the knees. Slowly bend the right knee and extend the left leg; maintaining continuous movement, slide the body to the left, flexing the left knee and extending the right leg.
Lower back, hamstrings, calves, and shoulders	Pelvic rock—Facing the wall, bring your legs out to the front of the body. The legs can be anywhere from shoulder-width apart to completely together. The feet can be as high up the wall as is comfortable. The toes, knees, and hips are in alignment. Visualizing the pelvis as a bowl, flex the knees and rock the pelvic bowl in toward the wall, filling the bowl with water. Gently rock back to the original position, dumping all the water out of your pelvic bowl toward the bottom of the pool. This should feel wonderful; if you experience any discomfort, you are exceeding your appropriate range of motion.

You are the creator of your own personalized deep-water workout. The formula presented for the workout is effective, but the time spent in each phase should reflect how you are feeling, your current level of fitness, and your exercise program goals. The deep-water exercises presented can also be used as a supplement to your shallow-water movement phrases by adding them to the aerobic portion of your workout. As you comply with the basic requirement of exercising aerobically at least three times per week for 20 to 60 minutes, you will be on your way to achieving your fitness goals. In the words of the famous UCLA basketball coach John Wooden, "Do not let what you cannot do interfere with what you can do."

Deep-Water Workout Equipment

In the deep-water workout program, the only aquatic equipment absolutely necessary is a flotation device to assist in suspending the body upright and allowing the head to remain comfortably above the water. As we all have different needs and body types, choose a belt or vest that works best for you.

If you desire to vary your workouts or increase the intensity, there is a multitude of resistance equipment you can purchase. Be sure you do not compromise your body alignment or exercise technique when adding resistance equipment to your workout. The equipment that can be added are webbed gloves, Hydro-Tone Bells and/or Boots, Hydro-Fit and other brand cuffs, and an aqua belt (designed to increase upper-body resistance), which will fit over or under a flotation device. (See Appendix F for a list of vendors selling aquatic buoyancy vests, belts, and resistance equipment.)

Special Situations

The beauty of deep-water workouts is that anyone, using the appropriate flotation device in the nearly weightless environment of the water, can participate and reap some benefits. There are special situations, however, where certain adjustments or modifications must be made. These situations may include but are not limited to conditions of pregnancy, rehabilitation from an injury, and the use of medications. Chapter 9 described modifications and guidelines for persons with such special needs.

For arthritic exercisers, deep-water exercising may be better than shallow-water exercising since in this environment zero impact is placed on the musculoskeletal system. Arthritic exercisers appear to gain the best results when exercising in water that is 90° to 94° F. Consult with your physician before beginning a deep-water exercise program.

Persons involved in cardiac rehabilitation programs and those with serious lower-back problems are also advised to consult a physician before embarking on a deep-water exercise program. In most cases, deep-water workouts are ideal for those with lower-back problems due to the zero-impact environment. It is quite common to diminish or even eliminate lower-back pain with deep-water exercising. Be sure to practice proper body alignment and safe exercise techniques to reap the benefits from this exercise program.

Checklist: Precautions

1. Execute proper body alignment—this is paramount for a safe and effective workout!
2. Breathe normally through the mouth and nose.
3. Listen to your body at all times and respond accordingly.
4. Work at your own pace and at your own level of intensity.
5. Don't try to keep up with your friend, partner, or instructor!
6. Use smooth, flowing movements that involve both arms and legs simultaneously.
7. Vary movement patterns.
8. Don't create stress on your body by hyperextending the joints.
9. Keep your body warm throughout your workout. Don't let your body become chilled.
10. Stretch to where you feel tension, not pain.
11. Exercise with a buddy if you're not in a class.
12. Have fun! Laugh and don't take yourself too seriously.

Summary

1. Deep-water workouts allow a person to add another dimension to his/her aquatic exercise program and work out in a zero-impact environment.
2. Always use proper body alignment in your deep-water workouts.
3. Understand and accept that exhaustion has no place in any exercise program: don't overdo it or push too hard.
4. Deep-water workouts can be used by athletes to enhance performance in their sport or for rehabilitation from an injury.
5. Additional resistance equipment can be added to your deep-water workout to increase the intensity. Do not compromise proper technique or your body position to increase the intensity.
6. Since exercising in deep water imposes zero impact on the exerciser, these activities are particularly well-suited for arthritic exercisers.
7. Have fun with your workouts!

CHAPTER 12

Training Alternatives and Variations

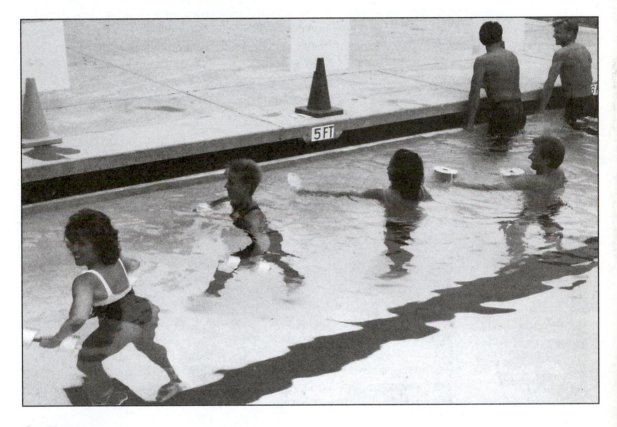

Outline

Cross Training

Cross training is a term applied to the use by athletes and avid exercisers of a variety of activities in order to avoid overuse injuries and/or boredom, to perfect different movement forms, or to add resistance to an activity. One example of the use of cross training on an alternating schedule would be the exercise program of a person who jogs on land Monday, Wednesday, and Friday, and executes a jogging workout in a swimming pool Tuesday, Thursday, and Saturday. An example of more varied cross training would be the program of an individual who jogs two days a week, plays basketball two days a week and racquetball one day a week, and takes a dance-exercise aerobics class and an aqua aerobics class one day a week.

Interval Training

Interval training combines segments of high-intensity aerobic training with periods of low-intensity aerobic training or rest. The heart rate remains in the target zone, but fluctuates between the minimum and maximum levels for the individual. For advanced participants, the high-intensity period might be as long as three minutes, followed by a one-and-a-half minute low-intensity period. For less-advanced persons, the high-intensity period might be one to one-and-a-half minutes long, followed by a three- to four-minute low-intensity period. The times can be adjusted based on the ability of the exerciser, and can increase progressively as the individual improves.

Interval training will provide you with a cardiovascular–respiratory workout as well as improved muscular endurance. Interval training is integrated into the aerobic portion of the aquatic exercise workout. Your workout must still begin with a thermal warm-up, pre-stretches, and cardiovascular–respiratory warm-up, followed by the aerobic portion of the workout. The workout then continues with muscular strength and endurance training, and the final cool-down and stretch periods. Interval training will provide variety for you during your aquatic workout.

Examples of Interval Training Activities

1. Walk at a brisk pace through the entire shallow area of the pool three times. Then go to the side of the pool, hang on to the pool edge or gutter, and try quickly to climb up and down the side wall of the pool five times. Repeat the entire exercise three times.
2. Slide through the entire shallow area of the pool two times. Then go to the side of the pool and hold on to the gutter or edge of the pool. Jump on the bottom of the pool and try to bring your fanny up in the air and then straddle jump, trying to get your feet up near the gutter area.
3. Repeat Exercise 2 above, but jog through the water instead of slide.
4. Run through the shallow area of the pool four times. Each time stop in the shallow area of the pool and jump out of the water as high and as fast as you can. Stretch your arms up overhead on each jump.

Interval training
example #1

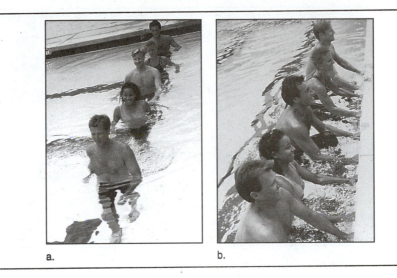

a.   b.

Interval training example #4

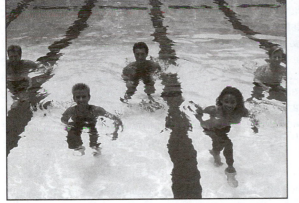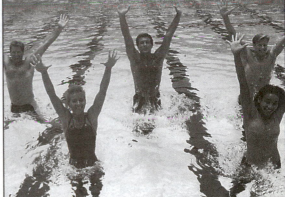

a.   b.

Circuit Training

Circuit training alternates between segments of cardiovascular–respiratory training and muscular strength training. Circuit training is used after a proper warm-up and stretch have taken place. A 20- to 45-minute circuit training segment can follow the warm-up, and the workout should then end with cool-down and stretch segments to promote flexibility. The circuit would consist of strength stations alternating with aerobic intervals of one to five minutes.

Circuit training techniques can also be integrated into the aerobic portion of an aqua aerobics class by dividing that section into two 10- to 15-minute sections. The first section would be traditional aqua aerobic movements, and the second section would be the circuit training segment. Circuit training integrated into a traditional aqua aerobics class can provide the exerciser with variety.

Circuit training

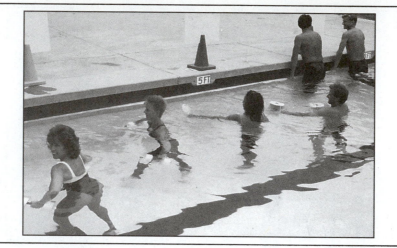

Bench-Stepping Aquatic Exercise

A recent addition to the aquatic exercise arena is the use of a small bench (6 to 10 inches high) placed in the shallow end of the water, upon which the exerciser steps up and down in various patterns. This bench-stepping type of aerobic activity has been used in dance-exercise aerobics classes for a number of years, but only recently was added to the aquatic exercise environment. Problems that prevented immediate adaptation of bench stepping were that several of the brands of benches on the market floated when placed in the water, jiggled when the water was turbulent, and/or gradually disintegrated from the chemicals used in pools. Now there are several companies that produce benches that do not float, remain stable, and do not disintegrate from the water, thus allowing aquatic exercisers to add bench-stepping activities to their workouts. (See Appendix F for brands.)

Bench-stepping activities offer additional variety for the aerobic portion of your workout. The resistance and cushioning properties of the water, combined with the use of a bench, provide a progressively challenging and enjoyable method to alternate with the types of movements used during the aerobic portion of a traditional aquatic workout. An aquatic workout using bench-stepping aerobic activities will still begin with a thermal warm-up, a stretch, and a cardiovascular–respiratory warm-up. Then the bench-stepping aerobic activities will begin and continue in a progressive manner for 20 to 30 minutes. The aerobic portion of the workout must be followed by a traditional cool-down and a flexibility section.

The bench-stepping aerobic activities consist of stepping up onto the bench and back down onto the floor of the pool in a variety of directions, as well as locomotor movements around the bench. The movements must alternate the leading leg stepping up and down to work the muscles in both legs equally. Begin your bench-stepping aquatic workout in waist-deep water. Progression in difficulty is accomplished by gradually moving the bench to deeper water and by increasing the intricacy of the stepping patterns used. The deeper the water, the greater the resistance through which your body will be moving. To assist your balance, dumbbell-type flotation devices can be held in each hand for sta-

Bench-stepping

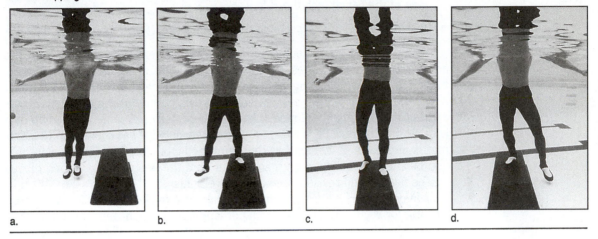

a.   b.   c.   d.

bility. Once you master balancing yourself, the dumbbells can be used as resistance equipment when arm movement patterns are added to the legwork as well as webbed gloves.

Sample Bench-Stepping Movements

Begin facing the width of the bench. Stand with your chest parallel to the side edge of the bench. (Key: R = right and L = left.)

- Step up R, up L, down R, down L.
  Step up L, up R, down L, down R.

- Step up R, lift a straight L leg up behind you, pull the L leg in next to the R, and step on the bench. Step down R, step down L. Repeat beginning on L foot.

- Walk around the bench clockwise.

- With your R side to the edge of the bench, step up R, step up L, then step down to the R side of the bench with your R foot and then L foot so that your L side will be to the edge of the bench. With your L side to the edge of the bench, step up L, step up R, step to the L side of the bench with your L foot so your R side will be to the edge of the bench and then step down on your R foot.

- Jog clockwise around the bench.

- Facing the width of the bench so that your chest is parallel to the side edge, step up R, step up L, step down R, step down L. Repeat in reverse.

- Slide all the way around the bench.

- Begin with your right shoulder to the side of the bench. Step up onto R, step up L, then step down to the R side of the bench on the R foot. Step down on the L foot to the L side of the bench. Step up L, step up R. Step down to the L side of the bench with L foot, step down to the R side of the bench with R foot to straddle the bench. Step up R foot, step up L foot, step down to the L side of the bench with L foot, and then step down on the L side of the bench with the R foot.

- Jog forward all the way around the bench. Repeat in the opposite direction.

Any combination of step-up and step-down movements will work with the aquatic bench-step activities. Use your imagination and create movement combinations that are challenging to you. Once you have become proficient at bench-stepping activities you can add interesting and challenging arm movements to each stepping phrase. Also, the step up can become a step hop or a leap. At first, however, it is wiser to concentrate on your basic lower-body movements and balance. Remember that dumbbell-type flotation devices will help you balance while stepping up and down onto the bench, and webbed gloves can be used to add resistance to arm movements.

Many people like to use bench-step aquatic workouts as a form of cross training for regular aquatic workouts or land-based bench-step workouts.

Aqua Walking

Aqua walking is a popular type of workout for many people. Walking through the water forcefully can increase your heart rate and add variety to the type of aquatic exercise movements you perform during an aerobic workout. An aquatic workout using aqua-walking aerobic activities will still begin with a thermal warm-up, a stretch, and a cardiovascular–respiratory warm-up. Then walking aerobic activities will begin and continue in a progressive manner for 20 to 30 minutes. The aerobic portion of the workout must be followed by a traditional cool-down and a flexibility section.

Adding the use of resistance equipment to the hands, arms, and/or legs will greatly increase the intensity of the workout. Resistance equipment that can be added to the hands include paddles, webbed gloves, Hydro-Tone Bells, and foam dumbbells. Using Hydro-Tone Bells will cause the workout's intensity to increase the most dramatically. Resistance equipment can also be worn or strapped onto the legs to increase the intensity of the workout. A variety of companies produce foam "anklet"-type resistance equipment that can be strapped onto the ankles to increase the resistance of the legs moving through the water. The pieces of equipment that will provide the most resistance to leg movements are Hydro-Tone Boots.

Aqua Jogging

Aqua jogging is also popular with many people as an aerobic workout. Jogging in water provides additional resistance that the exerciser must overcome, as well as a lower-impact environment than land jogging. As with the other variations of an aquatic workout, you must begin with a thermal warm-up, followed by a stretch and a cardiovascular–respiratory warm-up. Then you may begin jogging through the water and continue in a progressive manner for 20 to 30 minutes. The aerobic portion of the workout must be followed by a traditional cool-down and flexibility section.

When first jogging in the water, do not be concerned with how far you go during your aerobic workout, although you could eventually use distance as a measure of your increasing strength and endurance. Jogging can be done in any direction, in any formation, and with the use of any arm movements. Some people like to perform aquatic jogging at their own pace, without regard to any type of choreographic phrasing or musical coordination. Instead of being concerned with whether your jogging pace matches the tempo of the music, the aquatic jogger may listen to background "muzak" or may work in silence.

As with aqua walking, the same resistance equipment can be worn on the body to increase the intensity of the workout.

Sport-Specific Aquatic Exercises

Athletes have begun practicing sports activities in water to perfect their skills. In the aquatic environment the movements are cushioned, which reduces the risk of injury. Also, the athlete is working against the additional resistance of the water. Performing sports skills in the water forces the movements to be slower due to the water's resistance. These extra seconds per movement allow the athlete to:

1. "Feel" his/her body parts in "freeze frame."
2. Provide more time for analysis and personal feedback.
3. Promote opportunities to correct movements.

Drilling skills specific to the sport performed in the water will also add variety to an athlete's workout schedule.

Sports that can be practiced in the water are baseball, basketball, cross-country skiing, racquet sports, sprinting, cheerleading, and gymnastics. Examples of drills that can be used in the water for some of these sports follow.

Baseball Swing

Use an old baseball bat and practice swinging it in the water. Try full swings, bunting, and switch-hitting.

Baseball swing

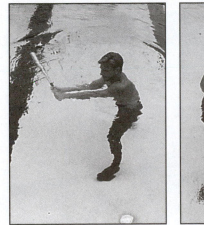 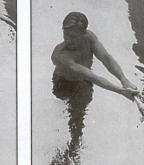

a.   b.

Basketball Jump Shot

Take a training partner and an old basketball to the pool. Practice your jump shot, jumping as high as you can in the water. Shoot toward your partner. When your partner returns the ball to you, jump high to receive it and shoot again.

Basketball jump shot

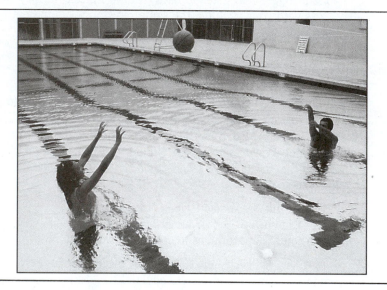

Tennis, Badminton, and Racquetball

Take an old racquet into the pool and execute your swings in the water. The water will give you the resistance necessary to improve strength and endurance in the muscles used specifically in your sport. Concentrate on using good form. Since the water slows your movements down, you can perfect your strokes.

Tennis swing

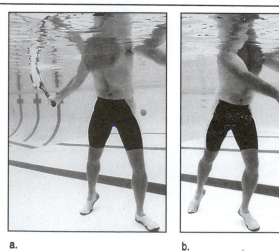

a.   b.

Sprinting on a Tether

In water, you can perfect your sprinting technique without the risk of injury by using a tether. Attach one end of an elastic tether around your waist and the other end to the ladder or side of the pool. The tether will allow you to lean forward into the proper sprinting position. Working in chest-deep water sprint in place, concentrating on perfect arm action and proper knee lift. Execute your interval training workout based on time rather than distance. An example is to run five 45-second sprints to approximate five 300-meter sprints.

Cheerleading

Practice jumps in the water. The resistance of the water will improve your land performance as well as cushion your landings, thus reducing the risk of injuries. Practice pyramid activities in the water in the initial stages to avoid injury.

Checklist: Training Alternatives

1. List activities you might like to use for cross training.
2. Are you currently using the technique of cross training?
3. List two examples of interval-training activities.
4. Describe circuit training.
5. Try bench stepping activities in the water if you have a bench available to you.
6. Practice aqua walking through the shallow end of the pool and see if you can elevate your heart rate to your target zone.
7. After warming up properly, time yourself jogging through the shallow end of the pool. Practice this for several days and see if your time decreases.
8. If you participate in a sport, think of skills in your sport that you could practice in the water. Try them out in the water for several days and see if your land-based performance improves.

Summary

1. *Cross training* is a term applied to the use by athletes and avid exercisers of a variety of activities in order to avoid overuse injuries and/or boredom.
2. Cross training offers the exerciser motivation to perfect different movement forms.
3. Interval training combines segments of high-intensity aerobic training with periods of low-intensity aerobic training.

4. Circuit training alternates between segments of cardiovascular–respiratory training and muscular strength training.

5. A recent addition to aquatic exercise is the use of a small bench (8 to 10 inches high) placed in the shallow end of the pool, which the exerciser steps up onto and down from in various patterns. This type of exercising is called aquatic bench-step aerobics.

6. Walking through the water forcefully (or aqua walking) can increase your heart rate and add variety to the type of aquatic-exercise movements you choose to perform during an aerobic workout.

7. Aqua jogging is another popular movement form that many people use as an aerobic workout. Water provides additional resistance to the jogger and offers a lower-impact environment than that on land.

8. Athletes have begun practicing sports activities in the water to perfect their skills—this activity has been called "sport-specific training." In the aquatic environment the movements are cushioned, which reduces the risk of injury and offers the athlete additional resistance while practicing a sports skill.

CHAPTER 13

Selecting an Aqua Aerobics Class

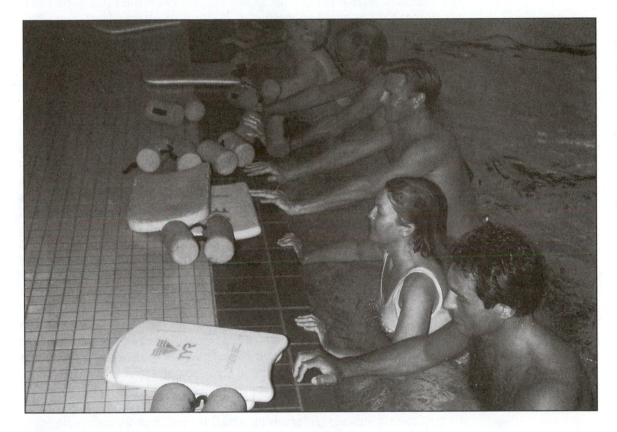

Outline

What to Look for in an Instructor

When you think about signing up for an aqua aerobics class, you probably will wonder where to begin. There are many teachers to choose from and many places to take classes. Some people erroneously think that if the instructor looks good, then that person must be a good instructor. Unfortunately, many establishments employ instructors based on their appearance instead of their qualifications. After reading this chapter, you will know the right questions to ask to seek out a qualified instructor. If you take classes from a qualified instructor, you will be able to get the most out of your workout.

Characteristics of a Good Instructor

Good instructors teach with enthusiasm and genuine concern for their students. They come to class well-prepared to teach and arrive in ample time to set up the pool area and begin the class on time. An instructor should always start a class promptly and finish on schedule. Before the series of classes begins, a good instructor explains the goals of his/her aqua aerobics class, how and why to take your pulse, and how to determine your target heart range. A good aqua aerobics instructor should be a role model, a person who is fit and who lives a healthy lifestyle. (This does not necessarily mean that your instructor should look like he/she walked off the cover of a magazine—not all good instructors look like models or movie stars.) Other very important characteristics of a good instructor are that he/she has a professional affiliation with an educational resource organization and demonstrates a commitment to continuing education. Also, your instructor should have a fitness certificate or equivalent certification from a university or a private certifying organization.

It is very important for your safety that your instructor has an appropriate knowledge base in exercise physiology and injury prevention and demonstrates only safe and effective exercise techniques. Other very important certifications that your instructor should have include cardiopulmonary resuscitation (CPR), first aid, and emergency water safety skills. Additional important questions to ask the pool management are: Is there a lifeguard on duty? If not, is the instructor proficient in lifesaving/lifeguarding skills? Is there appropriate rescue equipment and an emergency telephone available on the pool deck?

Some questions for you to consider yourself include: Does the instructor conduct the class in a nonintimidating and noncompetitive manner? Is he/she there for a personal workout or for *you*? Is the instructor conscious of how the environment is affecting the class? Is the air too hot or too cold? Is the water too hot or too cold? Is the music too loud? Are people bumping into one another? A good instructor will be cognizant of these factors and make the appropriate adjustments. The instructor should be aware of the fatigue level of the class and look for signs of overexertion. Similarly, individuals who appear not to be working hard enough need to be encouraged.

The Aqua Aerobics Class Format

Every instructor has his/her own unique style, and that's good! However, all classes should follow the same basic formula. First, there should be a seven- to ten-minute warm-up that includes all major muscle groups and avoids ballistic stretches. Following the warm-up is the aqua aerobics section of class, which lasts 15 to 30 minutes, depending on the length of the class. During this time, there should be a gradual build-up, a sustained high-intensity level, and a gradual decrease in intensity. Finally, it is important to have the post-aqua aerobics cool-down, where intensity gradually decreases so as not to shock the system with a sudden change of pace. Your instructor should guide you to check your pulse rate about five minutes into the aqua aerobics section and near the end of it. There should also be a post-aerobic recovery check two to three minutes after cool-down or at the end of the class.

The aqua aerobic exercises used by an instructor should flow smoothly and skillfully from one movement to another, as should one section of class to the next. The cues given by the instructor should be easily understood, and the movements should be challenging and keep your interest. Too much time spent on one activity without variation leads to boredom. A good instructor changes the movements frequently, yet allows enough repetition so you can eventually master them all.

A good class also includes about 10 to 15 minutes of exercises to strengthen the muscles of the arms, chest, shoulders, abdomen, back, legs, buttocks, and hips. A five-minute cool-down for these strengthening exercises includes static stretches for every muscle group worked.

Selecting a Facility

A good facility or club makes you feel positive about yourself and want to return to work out again soon. A well-run facility is concerned about your welfare and not only your membership, as mentioned previously. An important question to ask the facility is at what temperatures the pool and the air are kept. Ideally, the pool should be kept at 82° to 84° for aqua aerobics classes, and the air approximately 3° higher than the water. If the air temperature is not kept in this range, then the exerciser's discomfort increases as body parts exposed to cooler air will cause the body's core temperature to cool down very quickly. Unfortunately, however, most schools, public pools, and health clubs tend to keep the water in their pools closer to 80° to attempt to meet the needs of all of their aquatic exercisers—long-distance swimmers as well as aqua aerobics participants.

A qualified, concerned facility director hires only qualified instructors and makes sure that they are familiar with the equipment and safety skills. A good facility maintains a clean, hygienic environment. The pool area, showers, restrooms, and locker rooms should be clean and well-maintained. The temperature should be well-regulated in the pool, shower room, and dressing area.

If the facility has weight equipment, the area should be effectively supervised by qualified leaders. The equipment should be well-maintained and in good working order. Policies should be established and enforced to allow all members easy access to the equipment. If the facility has weight-training equipment, there should be someplace where you can keep a log of your progress filed for easy accessibility each time you exercise.

When selecting the facility, be sure to check its schedule of classes. Does it offer classes at times you can attend? (If it doesn't, the facility won't be of much use to you.) Does it demonstrate a willingness to adapt to the clients' requests for different time slots, more classes, and a variety of offerings (e.g., beginning, intermediate, and advanced aqua aerobics classes)? Are other services available, such as nutrition counseling, physical therapy, massage, a pro shop, social activities, and a referral network of physicians in case of injury? Is the facility convenient to your home or work? Does it provide childcare facilities? Does the membership fee fit into your budget?

All of these considerations must be well-evaluated when selecting a facility. Choose the facility that best meets your needs. If you don't, you may find that you have joined a club you won't really use. So take time now to investigate the facility before you join—it will save you money and aggravation in the future.

Checklist: Selecting a Facility

1. Is the facility conveniently located?
2. Are there classes given at the times you desire?
3. Is the pool well-maintained and the water kept at a good temperature?
4. Are there weight-training facilities?
5. What are the qualifications of the instructors for aqua aerobics, weight training, and all other classes?
6. Are there other facilities, such as a physical therapy area or a pro shop?
7. What social activities are offered (e.g., socials, dances, trips, tournaments)?
8. Can you afford the membership fee?

Summary

1. Your most important consideration is the instructor you choose for your class.
2. A good instructor:
   - Is certified by an accredited organization and/or is university-trained.
   - Holds a CPR (cardiopulmonary resuscitation) card, is trained in first aid, has emergency water safety skills, and is concerned about your safety.
   - Arrives on time and begins on time.
   - Is clear and thorough about the goals of the class.
   - Assists you in finding your target heart rate.
   - Conducts the class in a non-intimidating manner.
3. Characteristics of an effective class include:
   - Ten minutes of warm-up.

- Twenty to 30 minutes of aqua aerobic work that keeps you at your target heart rate.
- A three- to five-minute aqua aerobic cool-down.
- Approximately 10 to 15 minutes of strength development and toning.
- Five minutes of cool-down activities and flexibility following the strengthening exercises.

4. A facility should have:

- A well-maintained pool, with water temperature kept between 82° and 84°.
- Air temperature in the pool area 3° above the pool temperature.
- Clean and well-maintained shower and dressing areas.
- Classes at convenient times.

CHAPTER 14

Purchasing Media for Personal Use

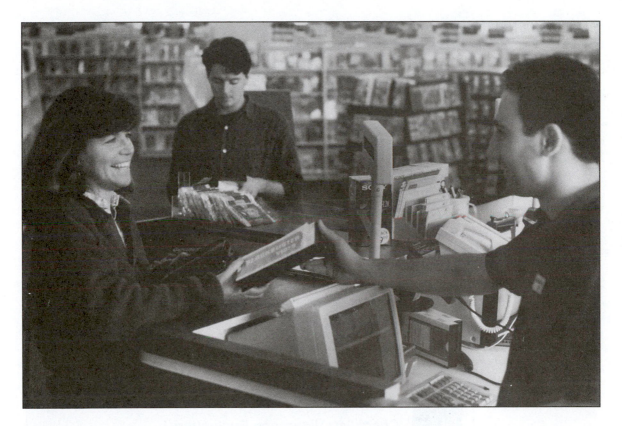

Outline

You may find that occasionally you have to miss an aqua aerobics class and you'll need to work out at your home pool or in a hotel/motel pool if you are traveling. At home, you may be able to place your videotape equipment and television monitor next to your pool so that you can work out at home, but this would be rather difficult to accomplish at most hotel/motel pools. To prepare for one of these situations you could buy a videotape (for home use) or music (to use at home or when traveling) to motivate you through a workout when you can't attend a class. Here are some guidelines for buying your media.

Selecting a Videotape

There are numerous aqua aerobics workout videotapes on the market from which to choose. The videotapes vary in ability level and style. For the most part, however, these home video workouts attempt to offer you a safe, effective, informative exercise program that you can execute in any shallow pool. Some videos simply present the exercise material, while others give you extensive scenery and elaborate camera angles. Though the content of a videotape is most important, an aesthetically well-done tape helps maintain your interest. Before you purchase a videotape, preview or rent it so that you can evaluate whether it meets your needs.

Evaluating a Videotape

In evaluating a videotape for purchase, rate the following five areas as they relate to your needs: instructor technique, balance and flow of the class, safety, technical proficiency of the production, and the overall effectiveness of the videotape for your purposes.

Checklist: Videotape Evaluation

After viewing the videotape, check the *yes* or *no* column for each question in the chart on the following page. Once you have completed the checklist, add up your *yes* responses and your *no* responses. If you have significantly more *yes* responses, the videotape is acceptable.

Videotape Evaluation	Yes	No
Instructor Technique		
1. Does the instructor give adequate cues to guide you into the movements?		
2. Can you follow the movements presented?		
3. Do you like the choreography?		
4. Are the transitions smooth?		
Class Balance		
1. Does the class include all five parts of a good lesson: warm-up, aqua aerobics, aqua aerobic cool-down, strength and flexibility, and a final cool-down?		
2. Is the time allotted to each section of the class properly balanced? Aqua warm-up: 7 to 10 minutes. Aqua aerobics: 15 to 30 minutes. Aqua aerobic cool-down: 5 minutes. Strengthening and toning: 10 to 15 minutes. Final cool-down and flexibility: 5 minutes.		
3. Is the entire body worked out in the routine?		
Safety Information		
1. Does the instructor discuss proper body alignment and/or proper execution of each exercise?		
2. Are the demonstrations executed with proper body alignment?		
3. Is there an accompanying guidebook that discusses exercise precautions?		
4. Is time allotted to check your heart rate?		
Technical Proficiency		
1. Are the camera angles appropriate for you to understand the movement?		
2. Do the camera angles assist your learning or detract from it?		
3. Is it difficult to follow the movement because of the way it is photographed?		
4. Is the music well-recorded?		
5. Do you like the music?		
6. Is the cuing properly coordinated with the demonstration?		
Overall Effectiveness		
1. Does the videotape provide you with a model you can follow?		
2. Is the videotape presentation of the class motivating to you?		
3. Did you enjoy exercising to the tape?		
4. Did the tape provide you with the workout you need?		
Totals		
Did you have more *yes* responses or *no* responses?		

After evaluating a videotape, review the checklist. If the responses are mostly positive, the tape should work for you. If the responses are mostly negative, keep reviewing videotapes until you find one that meets your needs.

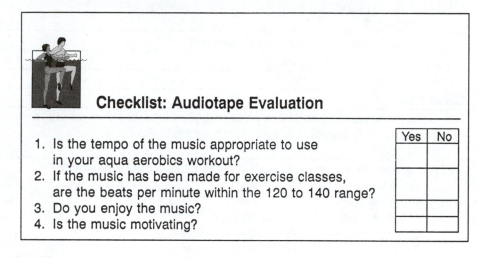

Checklist: Audiotape Evaluation

	Yes	No
1. Is the tempo of the music appropriate to use in your aqua aerobics workout?		
2. If the music has been made for exercise classes, are the beats per minute within the 120 to 140 range?		
3. Do you enjoy the music?		
4. Is the music motivating?		

Summary

1. It is nice to have a videotape or an audiotape to exercise with when you cannot make it to an aqua aerobics class or when you are traveling.
2. There are several aqua aerobics videotapes on the market for home exercise use. Preview any tape before you purchase it.
3. Evaluate the videotape you are considering purchasing for quality in the following areas: instructor technique, balance, safety, technical proficiency, and overall effectiveness.
4. Audiotapes are available for purchase with music adjusted to the appropriate tempo for aqua aerobics. Listen to an audiotape before you buy it, paying close attention to the appropriateness of the tempo, sound quality, and musical selections.

CHAPTER 15

Becoming an Instructor

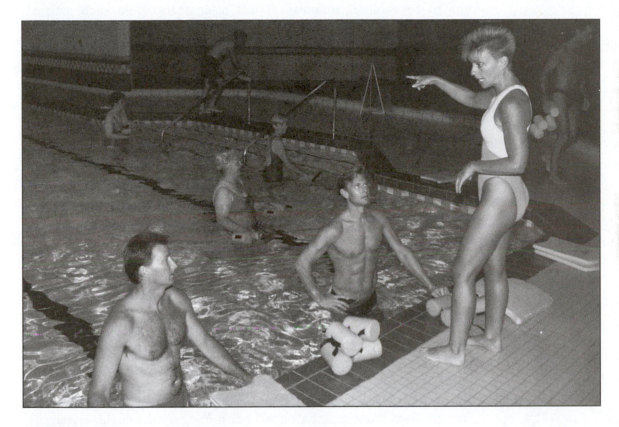

Outline

Where to Study to Become an Instructor
Checklist: Do I Want to Be an Instructor?
Summary

Many people who have taken aquatic exercise classes for a long time wonder what it takes to become an instructor. To become an instructor, you must first enjoy aqua aerobics. Second, you must be in good physical condition. Third, you must study exercise physiology, anatomy and kinesiology, nutrition and weight control, components of teaching aquatic exercise, water safety, and first aid and cardiopulmonary resuscitation. Finally, you must enjoy working with and helping people.

There is a movement in this country to require all aquatic exercise instructors to be certified. However, at this point, there is no such national mandate—the certification requirement rests with each state or private agency. At present, no state requires aquatic exercise instructors to be state or nationally certified. Many universities and private organizations offer fitness instructor certificates that are recognized by hiring agencies. Many firms require their instructors to be certified, which is a sign of a responsible organization. California recently adopted a law requiring a lifeguard to be on duty in addition to the instructor in all public pools. This law, however, does not apply to private pools or health clubs.

Consumers deserve to be taught by the very best persons available. If a class is taught by someone who is good looking but uneducated in aquatic exercise, the participants risk being injured and the organization risks a lawsuit. An aqua aerobics instructor who has not been adequately educated in the subject will often be unable to maintain class participation and/or enthusiasm. It is to a facility's advantage to hire well-trained instructors. Thus, if you would like to become an instructor, start taking classes and studying.

Where to Study to Become an Instructor

Many universities and colleges offer fitness instructor/aquatic exercise instructor certificates, with courses taught by well-educated and knowledgeable instructors. If your local university does not offer a certification program, your next source is a private agency. There are several private organizations offering aquatic exercise instructor certificates. The quantity and quality of instruction vary greatly from one organization to the next. You must thoroughly investigate the courses and the time you will spend in each. Make sure there are course offerings in the following subjects:

- Exercise physiology.
- Anatomy and kinesiology.
- Nutrition and weight control.
- Components of teaching aquatic exercise.
- Health screening, and modifying for individual variations.
- Water safety and rescue.
- First aid.
- Cardiopulmonary resuscitation.

Since there are several private organizations and colleges offering certificates, it may be hard to choose one. The decision is yours; you must study the options available to you. The largest and most recognized private agency certifications are offered through:

Aquatic Exercise Association
P. O. Box 497
Port Washington, WI 53074
(414) 284-3416

Aquatics Council
c/o American Alliance for Health, Physical Education,
     Recreation and Dance
1900 Association Drive
Reston, VA 22091
(703) 476-3400

Council for National Cooperation in Aquatics
901 W. New York Street
Indianapolis, IN 46202
(317) 638-4238

United States Water Fitness Association
P. O. Box 360133
9851-D Military Trail
Boynton Beach, FL 33436
(407) 732-9908

YMCA
101 N. Wacker Drive
Chicago, IL 60606
(312) 269-0516

If you do decide to become an aquatic exercise instructor, it is imperative that you take courses in the subjects mentioned. You want to do the best job you can as an instructor. To do that, you must be well-qualified and educated in all aspects of teaching aquatic exercise and water safety. Good luck to you!

Checklist: Do I Want to Be an Instructor?

1. Do I enjoy water exercise more than any other form of exercise?
2. Am I interested in leading and helping other people?
3. Am I good at motivating people?
4. Can I express myself well?
5. Do I have the desire, time, and money to go to school to study to become an instructor?
6. Am I willing to study for the courses necessary to become an instructor?

If you answered "yes" to these questions, you might well make a good instructor. Perhaps it is time for you to investigate the local schools and/or organizations that certify aquatic exercise instructors.

Summary

1. To become an aquatic exercise instructor, you must enjoy this kind of exercise and like to motivate people.
2. You need to be in good physical condition to be an aquatic exercise instructor.
3. You must study many subjects so that you will be well-prepared to be the best instructor you possibly can be. The subjects you will need to study include physiology, anatomy and kinesiology, nutrition and weight control, components of teaching aquatic exercise, water safety and rescue, and first aid and cardiopulmonary resuscitation.
4. Investigate the various places you can study to become an instructor. Both universities and private agencies offer programs.
5. Good luck to you, and happy exercising!

APPENDIX A

Student Health History

Before you begin your aqua aerobics program, it is important for your instuctor to know something about your history so that he/she can assist you, if necessary. Please fill out the form below and give it to your instructor by the second day of class.

Name   _____

Age   _____

Date   _____

Class
Section   _____

Doctor's
Name   _____

Doctor's
Phone
Number   _____

1.   Do you or does anyone in your immediate family have any of the following illnesses/conditions?

_____ asthma

_____ chest pain or discomfort

_____ diabetes

_____ emphysema

_____ epilepsy

_____ heart disease

_____ hypertension

_____ pregnancy

2.   Have you had any of the following within the past two years?

_____ back injury

_____ fracture

_____ general major surgery

_____ heart attack

_____ heart surgery

_____ sprain

_____ stroke

If so, please specify. _____

3. Do you smoke?

_____ Yes

_____ No

4.   Are you currently taking any medications?

____   Yes

____   No

  If yes, please specify. _____

5.   Are you currently under a doctor's care?

____   Yes

____   No

  If yes, please specify the reason. _____

6.   What is the date of your last physical examination?

_____

7.   According to your physician and/or charts, are you:

____   Overweight   If so, by how much?   _____

____   Underweight   If so, by how much?   _____

____   Normal

8.   Do you have any handicaps or current or chronic injuries that limit your physical abilities?

____   Yes

____   No

  If yes, please describe. _____

9.   What is your current swimming level?

____   Nonswimmer

____   Beginning swimmer

____   Intermediate to advanced swimmer

10.   How do you feel in shallow water?

____   Comfortable

____   Uncomfortable

11.   How do you feel in deep water?

____   Comfortable

____   Uncomfortable

12. What are your main goals in this class? (Rank them by placing a 1, 2, or 3 on the line next to your first, second, and third most important goals.)

_____ Tone muscles
_____ Build muscles
_____ Increase cardiovascular fitness
_____ Increase overall fitness
_____ Lose weight
_____ Gain weight
_____ Lose inches
_____ Stay the same
_____ Other (please describe) _____

13. Do you experience any back pain or discomfort on a regular basis?

_____ Yes
_____ No

14. Would you consider yourself to be under any stress now?

_____ Yes
_____ No
   If yes, please describe. _____
_____

15. What is your current activity level?

_____ Sedentary
_____ Somewhat active
_____ Active
_____ Very active

16. Please supply any additional information that might be helpful to your instructor.

_____
_____
_____
_____

Caloric Output for Exercising

ACTIVITY	*CALORIES/MINUTE	ACTIVITY	*CALORIES/MINUTE
BADMINTON	5.0- 7.5	GYMNASTICS	5.0
BASEBALL	2.4- 4.0	balancing	2.5
BASKETBALL	8.6	abdominal	3.0
BOWLING	4.0- 5.0	trunk bending	3.5
CANOE ROWING		hopping	6.5
slow (2-3mph)	2.0- 3.0	HANDBALL	10.0-13.3
moderate (4mph)	5.0- 7.0	HOCKEY	12.0-15.0
rapid (5-6 mph)	7.0- 8.0	HORSEBACK RIDING	3.0- 9.5
CLASSWORK (reading)	1.0- 2.0	JOGGING (slow)	10.0-15.0
CLIMBING	10.7- 13.2	RECLINING	1.5- 1.6
CYCLING		ROPE SKIPPING	12.0
5 mph	4.5	RUNNING	
9 mph	7.0	7 mph	10.0
13 mph	11.1	9 mph	11.0
DANCING		12 mph	14.5-19.4
slow	3.0	SHIVERING	5.0- 7.0
fast	4.0- 7.0	SKATING	
DOMESTIC WORK		ice	6.6
bed making	3.5	roller	7.8-13.0
dusting	2.5	SKIING (CROSS COUNTRY)	
ironing	1.7	moderate speed	10.0-16.0
meal preparation	2.5	maximum speed	15.0-19.0
cleaning floors	3.5	SLEEPING	1.0- 1.2
standing	2.6	SQUASH	10.0-11.0
typing	1.6	SWIMMING	
washing	2.6	breaststroke	11.0
DRESSING	1.5- 2.0	backstroke	11.5
DRIVING A CAR	2.0	crawl	14.0
EATING	2.0	TALKING	1.0- 1.2
FARM CHORES	2.0- 3.0	TENNIS	7.1- 7.5
FENCING	5.0	table	5.0
FOOTBALL		WALKING	
touch	8.9	2 mph	2.5
tackle	12.0	3 mph	3.5
GOLF	5.0	5 mph	5.5
		up stairs	10.0-12.0
		WRESTLING	7.0- 9.0

*3500 Calories equals 1 pound

Energy Equivalents

Minutes of participation in the activities listed at right needed to expend the calorie energy of the foods listed below.

	Calorie content	Reclining	Walking	Bicycle Riding	Swimming	Running
Beverages						
Carbonated, 8 oz. glass	106	82	20	13	9	5
Ice cream soda, chocolate	255	196	49	31	23	13
Malted milkshake, chocolate	502	386	97	61	45	26
Milk, 8 oz. glass	166	128	32	20	15	9
Milk, skim, 8. oz. glass	81	62	16	10	7	4
Milkshake, chocolate	421	324	81	51	38	22
Beer, 8 oz. glass	114	88	22	14	10	6
Wine, 3 1/2 oz. glass	84	65	16	10	8	4
Desserts						
Cake, 2 layer	356	274	68	43	32	18
Cookie, chocolate chip	51	39	10	6	5	3
Doughnut	151	116	29	18	13	8
Ice cream, 1/6 Qt.	193	148	37	24	17	10
Gelatin, with cream	117	90	23	14	10	6
Pie, apple, 1/6	377	290	73	46	34	19
Sherbet, 1/6 Qt.	177	136	34	22	16	9
Strawberry shortcake	400	308	77	49	36	21
Fruit & Fruit Juices						
Apple, large	101	78	19	12	9	5
Banana, small	88	68	17	11	8	4
Orange, medium	68	52	13	8	6	4
Peach, medium	46	35	9	6	4	2
Apple juice, 8 oz. glass	118	91	23	14	10	6
Orange juice, 8 oz. glass	120	92	23	15	11	6
Tomato juice, 8 oz. glass	48	37	9	6	4	2
Meats						
Bacon, 2 strips	96	74	18	12	9	5
Ham, 2 slices	167	128	32	20	15	9
Pork chop, loin	314	242	60	38	28	16
Steak, T-bone	235	184	45	29	21	12

Minutes of participation in the activities listed at right needed to expend the calorie energy of the foods listed below.	Calorie content	Reclining	Walking	Bicycle Riding	Swimming	Running
Miscellaneous						
Bread & butter, 1 slice	78	60	15	10	7	4
Cereal, dry 1/2 c. w/milk, sugar	200	154	38	24	18	10
French dressing, 1 tbsp.	59	45	11	7	5	3
Mayonnaise, 1 tbsp.	92	71	18	11	8	5
Pancake, with syrup	124	95	24	15	11	6
Spaghetti, 1 serving	396	305	76	48	35	20
Cottage cheese, 1 tbsp.	27	21	5	3	2	1
Poultry & Eggs						
Chicken, fried 1/2 breast	232	178	45	28	21	12
Chicken "TV dinner"	542	217	104	66	48	28
Turkey, 1 slice	130	100	25	16	12	7
Egg, fried	110	85	21	13	10	6
Egg, boiled	77	59	15	9	7	4
Sandwiches & Snacks						
Club	590	454	113	72	53	30
Hamburger	350	269	67	43	31	18
Roast beef with gravy	430	331	83	52	38	22
Tunafish salad	278	214	53	34	25	14
Pizza, with cheese, 1/8	180	138	35	22	16	9
Potato chips, 1 serving	108	83	21	13	10	6
Cheddar cheese, 1 oz.	111	85	21	14	10	6
Seafood						
Clams, 6 medium	100	77	19	12	9	5
Cod, steamed, 1 piece	80	62	15	10	7	4
Crabmeat, 1/2 cup	68	52	13	8	6	4
Haddock, 1 piece	71	55	14	9	6	4
Halibut steak, 1/4 lb.	205	158	39	25	18	11
Lobster, 1 medium	50	38	10	6	4	3
Shrimp, french fried, 1 serv.	180	138	35	22	16	9
Vegetables						
Beans, green, 1 cup	27	21	5	3	2	1
Beans, canned, 1/2 cup	38	29	7	5	3	2
Carrot, raw	42	32	8	5	4	2
Lettuce, 3 large leaves	30	23	6	4	3	2
Peas, green, 1/2 cup	56	43	11	7	5	3
Potato, boiled, 1 medium	100	77	19	12	9	5
Spinach, fresh, 1/2 cup	20	15	4	2	2	1

SUGGESTED WEIGHT

HEIGHT[1]	WEIGHT IN POUNDS[2]	
	19 to 34 years	35 years and over
5'0"	97-128[3]	108-138
5'1"	101-132	111-143
5'2"	104-137	115-148
5'3"	107-141	119-152
5'4"	111-146	122-157
5'5"	114-150	126-162
5'6"	118-155	130-167
5'7"	121-160	134-172
5'8"	125-164	138-178
5'9"	129-169	142-183
5'10"	132-174	146-188
5'11"	136-179	151-194
6'0"	140-184	155-199
6'1"	144-189	159-205
6'2"	148-195	164-210
6'3"	152-200	168-216
6'4"	156-205	173-222
6'5"	160-211	177-228
6'6"	164-215	182-234

[1] Without shoes.

[2] Without clothes.

[3] The higher weights in the ranges generally apply to men, who tend to have more muscle and bone; the lower weights more often apply to women, who have less muscle and bone.

Adapted from
"Nutrition and Your Health: Dietary Guidelines for Americans," 3rd ed., 1990, U.S. Department of Agriculture, U.S. Department of Health and Human Services.

APPENDIX B

References: Books and Articles

Astrand, P., and K. Rodahl. *Textbook of Work Physiology*. New York: McGraw-Hill, 1977.

Casten, Carole, and Peg Jordan. *Aerobics Today*. St. Paul: West Publishing Company, 1990.

Chossek, Vicki, L. Delzeit, J. Lindle, R. Sova, and P. Windhorst. "Aquatic Concepts." Port Washington, WI: Aquatic Exercise Association, 1990.

Cooper, Kenneth. "The Riskiest Phase of Exercise." *Reebox Instructor News* Vol. 3, No. 5 (1990): 2.

Essert, Mary. "Water Exercise for Persons Who Have Arthritis." *The AKWA Letter* Vol. 4, No. 1 (1990): 4, 13.

Evans, B., K. Cureton, and J. Purvis. "Metabolic and Circulatory Responses to Walking and Jogging in Water." *Research Quarterly* 49 (1978): 4, 442-449.

Huey, Lynda. "Sport-Specific Water Training." *The AKWA Letter* Vol. 4, No. 2 (1990): 1, 11, 12.

Hydro-Tone International, "Hydro-Tone, The New Science of Total Fitness," 1989.

McArdle, W., F. Katch, and V. Katch. *Exercise Physiology*. Philadelphia: Lea & Febiger, 1990.

McCurdy, Mindy. "Cool Water Workout." *Shape* August, 1990: 64-73.

Midtlyng, Joanna. "Application of Selected Principles of Movement and Aquatic Skills to Water Exercise." *Water Exercise Teacher Syllabus*, Aquatic Council, American Alliance for Health, Physical Education, Recreation, and Dance, 1989.

Nicht, Sandra K. "Bench Aquatix, the No-Sweat Workout!" *The AKWA Letter* Vol. 4, No. 6 (1991): 1, 13.

Otis, Carol L. "When a Cooldown is Undesirable." *Women's Sports and Fitness* March, 1990: 8.

Sanders, Mary. "The Big Chill Is No Thrill . . . ." *The AKWA Letter* Vol. 4, No. 3 (1990): 1, 11-13.

Sova, Ruth. "Sample Bench Stepping Moves." *The AKWA Letter* Vol. 4, No. 6 (1991): 12.

Sova, Ruth, and Peg Windhorst. *Aquafit*, 1986.

Spitzer, Terry-Ann, J.R. Moore, D. Hopkins, and W. Hoeger. "A Comparison of Selected Training Responses to Water Aerobics and Low-Impact Aerobics." *The AKWA Letter* Vol. 4, No. 5 (1991).

"The Recommended Quantity and Quality of Exercise for Developing and Maintaining Cardiorespiratory and Muscular Fitness in Healthy Adults." *Medicine and Science in Sports and Exercise* April, 1990.

Thompson, Terri. "Aerobics." *Dance Teacher Now* March, 1988: 9-10.

Thornton, James S. "Hypothermia Shouldn't Freeze Out Cold-Weather Athletes." *The Physician and Sports Medicine* January, 1990: 109.

Vickery, S.R., K.J. Cureton, and J.L. Langstaff. "Heart Rate and Energy Expenditure During Aqua Dynamics." *The Physician and Sports Medicine* 11: 67-72.

Whitley, J., and L. Schoene. "Comparison of Heart Rate Responses: Water Walking versus Treadmill Walking." *Physical Therapy* 67 (1987): 1501-1504.

Wigglesworth, J.E., J.K. Edwards, A. Mikesky, and E. Evenbeck. "The Effect of Water Exercise on Various Parameters of Physical Fitness." *The AKWA Letter* Vol. 4, No. 3 (1990).

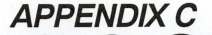

Perceived Exertion Chart Vendors

Fitness First
P.O. Box 251
Shawnee Mission, KS 66201
(913) 381-1983

Fitness Chart Series
3125 19th Street, Suite 305
Bakersfield, CA 93301
(805) 861-1100

Pro-Fit
P.O. Box 2339
Kirkland, WA 98083
(206) 823-4703

Pulse
2221 E. Somerset Drive
Salt Lake City, UT 84121

Pulselite
(800) 345-7857

Young & Gilman
107 N. Main
Lansing, KS 66043

APPENDIX D

Footwear

A variety of aquatic exercise shoes is available for purchase at sporting goods stores and discount stores. Additionally, the following companies produce and/or sell shoes designed specifically for aquatic exercise:

Hydro-Fit Incorporated
440 Charnelton
Eugene, OR 07401
(800) 346-7295

Omega Corporation
130 Condor Street
East Boston, MA 02128
(617) 569-3400

Sprint Rothhammer International, Inc.
P. O. Box 5579
Santa Maria, CA 93456
(800) 235-2156

Available Audiocassettes and Videocassettes

Audiocassette Sources

Aerobics Power Mix
Power Productions
P.O. Box 3812
Gaithersburg, MD 20878
(800) 777-BEAT

Aerobix Mix
In-Lytes Productions
614 Sherburn Lane
Louisville, KY 40207
(800) 243-PUMP

Medical and Sports Music Institute
P.O. Box 70681
Eugene, OR
(503) 344-5323 for technical inquiries
(503) 331-2819 to order

Pure Workout Music
Palmtree Productions
444 Lincoln Blvd., Suite 151
Venice, CA 90291

David Shelton Productions
P.O. Box 652
Layton, UT 84014
(800) 272-4311

Sprint Rothhammer International, Inc.
P.O. Box 5579
Santa Maria, CA 93456
(800) 235-2156

Stromberg Productions
253 Rhodes Ct.
San Jose, CA 95126
(408) 295-8393
(800) 82-TUNES

Supreme Audio
P.O. Box 50
Marlborough, NH 03455
(800) 445-7398

Videocassette Sources

AKWA Bookstore
Aquatic Exercise Association
P.O. Box 497
Port Washington, WI 53074
(414) 284-3416

Hydro-Fit Incorporated
440 Charnelton
Eugene, OR 97401
(800) 346-7295

Sprint Rothhammer
International, Inc.
P.O. Box 5579
Santa Maria, CA 93456
(800) 235-2156

Water Aerobics, Inc.
938 Utopia
San Antonio, TX 78223

Aquatic Vendors and Equipment

Aerobic Workbench offers a full-size reinforced fiberglass step bench for the water. Call (813) 391-7419. For a free brochure, send your name and address to P.O. Box 2575 / Largo, FL 34649.

Aquarius Health and Fitness Products, Inc., offers a water workout station. Call (800) 742-8449 or write Plaza 222 S. U.S. Hwy. 1, Suite 202 / Tequesta, FL 33469.

Aquarobics Division of AFA offers water hoops. Call (803) 235-4066.

Aqua-Source International offers Dux water weights. Call (800) 728-4157.

Aquatic Exercise Products offers Aquaflex Paddles. Call (800) 962-7574 or (415) 485-5323, or write 3070 Kerner Blvd., Unit 5 / San Rafael, CA 94901.

Bioenergetics, Inc., offers Wet Vest, a custom-made, fitted flotation vest that fastens around the torso; it is excellent for non-swimmers or individuals with physical limitations. The company also produces a special vest for the physically and mentally challenged. Prices for these products vary according to individual needs. Bioenergetics, Inc., also sells Wet Belt, a flotation belt made of a soft, pliable foam that contours to the body and fastens in front with velcro, as well as Wet Hands, webbed gloves made of soft lycra spandex that increase upper body resistance.

B-Wise Enterprise offers swim fitness bars. Call (800) 360-WISE.

Cardiostep offers a step bench for the water. Call (800) 800-2BFIT or write 282 Newbury St., Suite 14 / Boston, MA 02116.

D.K. Douglas offers Wet Wrap. Call (800) 334-9070.

Excel Sports Science offers Aqua-Jogger, a compressed foam flotation belt that fastens in front with a plastic buckle. Call (800) 922-9544.

Hydro-Fit, Inc., offers hand buoys, buoyancy/resistance cuffs, Wave Webs, Wet Belt, and aqua footwear. For a free color brochure call (800) 346-7295 or (503) 484-4361, or write 440 Charnelton St. / Eugene, OR 97401.

Hydro-Tone offers Hydro-Belt, a soft, closed-cell foam flotation belt that fastens around the midsection, as well as Hydro-Bells for upper body and Hydro-Boots for lower body training. Call (800) 622-TONE or (405) 948-7754 for a product catalog.

J&B Foam Fabricators offers Swim Pal Belt, Water Wafer, Hand Bars, Swim Bars, and much more. For a free catalog call (800) 621-FOAM or write P.O. Box 144 / Ludington, MI 49431.

Nuvo Sport, Inc., offers the SpaBell Total Fitness System. For a free brochure call (703) 914-0637 or write 4954 Sauquoit Ln. / Annandale, VA 22003.

Speedo offers water shoes, weighted gloves, kickboards, exercise clothing, and much more. Call (800) 543-2763.

Sprint Rothhammer International, Inc., offers Sprint E.R. Belt, Sprint Cuffs, Sprint Water Gloves, shoes, and much more. Call (800) 235-2156 or write P.O. Box 5579 / Santa Maria, CA 93456.

SPRI Products, Inc., offers the SPRI Aqua Belt, designed to increase upper body resistance; it will fit over or under a flotation device. Call (800) 222-7774.

Sit and Reach Box

Construction

1. Using any sturdy wood or comparable construction material (¾ inch plywood or comparable construction material is recommended), cut the following pieces:
   2 pieces—12 in x 12 in.
   2 pieces—12 in. x 10 in.
   1 piece—12 in. x 21 in.
2. Assemble the pieces using nails or screws, and wood glue.
3. Inscribe the top panel with one centimeter gradations. It is crucial that the 23 centimeter line be exactly in line with the vertical plane against which the subject's feet will be placed.
4. Cover the apparatus with two coats of polyurethane sealer or shellac.
5. For convenience, a handle can be made by cutting a 1 in. x 3 in. hole in the top panel.
6. The measuring scale should extend from about 9 to 50 cm.

Constructing the sit and reach box

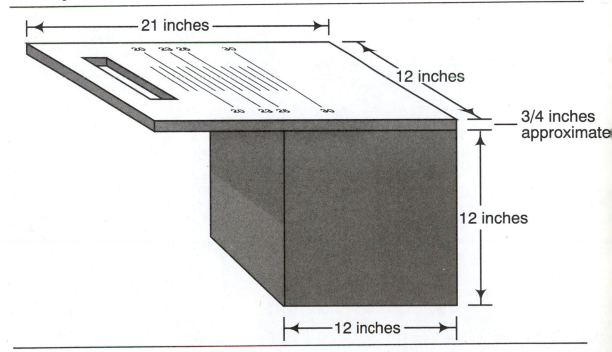

Aqua Aerobic Terms

Abduction is moving a body segment, such as an arm or a leg, away from the center line of the body (e.g., raising one's arms from a position alongside the body to an angle straight out from the shoulder).

Adduction is bringing the body segment back to the center line of the body (e.g., bringing the arms back toward the body from an angle straight out from the shoulder).

Aerobic refers to the use of oxygen by the body.

Aerobic capacity (cardiorespiratory endurance) is the ability of the body to remove oxygen from the air and transfer it, through the lungs and blood, to the working muscles.

Aerobic exercise is exercise for which the body is able to supply adequate oxygen to sustain performance for long periods of time.

Aerobics is a term applied to exercise that incorporates vigorous, continuous movements that, over a sustained period of time, require the body to utilize oxygen and increase the aerobic capacity of the body. It usually refers to dance-exercise-type classes that focus on fitness development.

Alignment refers to the correct positioning of the spine and the body parts. Alignment has postural implications (refers to how all the body parts line up).

Amino acids, the building blocks of protein, are organic compounds containing nitrogen, hydrogen, and carbon.

Anaerobic means without oxygen; it usually refers to the body's ability to perform short-spurt, high-energy activities, such as sprinting, without the need for oxygen replenishment.

Anatomy is described as the structural makeup of the human body.

Aqua aerobics/aquatic exercise is a form of exercise that incorporates a variety of movements in water, usually performed to motivating music. The purpose of this exercise is to provide the exerciser with an overall body-conditioning program.

Aqua physics is the application of the physical properties of water, including Sir Isaac Newton's laws of motion, to aquatic exercise. Newton's first law of motion states that an object remains either stationary or moves at a constant velocity unless acted upon by a force. The second law, the law of acceleration, states that the acceleration of an object depends upon its mass and on the applied force. The third law states that for every action there is an equal and opposite reaction.

Arteriosclerosis is the abnormal thickening or hardening of the arteries, which causes the inner artery walls to lose their elasticity.

Artery is the large vessel that carries oxygenated blood away from the heart to the body tissues.

Atherosclerosis is a general term for a disease that leads to the thickening and hardening of the inner layer of the artery wall due to fat deposits. It causes a decrease in the inner diameter of the artery.

Ballistic movements are those that are jerky, bouncy, explosive, and unsustained.

Ballistic stretching is bouncing under the misconception that one is stretching.

Basal metabolic rate is the sum total of energy required by all the physiologic processes required to maintain life; in other words, the number of calories burned to sustain life.

Blood pooling refers to a condition caused by ceasing vigorous exercise too abruptly so that blood remains in the extremities and may not be delivered quickly enough to the heart and brain.

Blood pressure refers to the amount of pressure the blood exerts against the walls of the arteries during each heart contraction and heart relaxation. Taking one's blood pressure measures the pressure of the blood in the arteries.

Body alignment is how the torso, limbs, spine, shoulders, head, etc., are positioned. Proper body alignment refers to the optimal placement and posture of the body during exercise to ensure safe, injury-free movement.

Body composition is the percentage of body fat to lean body mass (muscle, bone, cartilage, vital organs). Proper body composition is a part of overall fitness.

Buoyancy refers to the suspension of the body in the water. Archimedes' Principle states that an object will be suspended in a fluid by a force equal to the weight of the fluid displaced by the object.

Calorie is the common word used to refer to the kilocalorie. The kilocalorie is a measure of the value of foods that produce heat and energy in the body. One calorie is equal to the amount of heat required to raise the temperature of one gram of water one degree Centigrade.

Carbohydrate refers to organic compounds containing carbon, hydrogen, and oxygen. When broken down, carbohydrates are the main energy source for muscular work and one of the basic foodstuffs in a person's diet.

Cardiovascular efficiency refers to the ability of the body to deliver oxygen efficiently to all of its vital organs during the stress of exercise.

Carotid pulse is the pulse point located on the carotid artery in the neck, approximately one inch below the jawbone and next to the Adam's apple. It is the area commonly used for taking the heart rate during and following exercise, as it is easy to locate.

Cholesterol is a chemical compound found in animal fats and oils. High levels of cholesterol in the blood are often associated with a high risk of atherosclerosis.

Chronic refers to something persisting over a long period of time.

Concentric contraction is when the muscle shortens as it contracts. An example of this is the contraction that occurs when you lift up a curl bar to perform bicep curl exercises.

Conduction is the transfer of heat energy away from the body by substances with which it is in direct contact. Conduction can occur in any medium. Water's conductivity is 240 times greater than air, and therefore water is an excellent heat conductor.

Convection occurs when the body comes in contact with air or water that has a temperature lower than that of the body. When the air/water touches the body, the air/water is warmed and then carried away by a streaming movement.

Cool-down is the time allotted to allow the heart rate to lower gradually following aerobic exercise. Cool-down movements are usually slow and smooth.

Core temperature refers to the body's internal temperature.

Coronary arteries are the two main arteries of the heart in the aorta, just above the semilunar valves, where the oxygenated blood leaves the left ventricle. They are the major arteries responsible for carrying blood to the heart muscle.

Cross training is a term applied to the use of a variety of fitness activities and movement forms by athletes and avid exercisers to avoid overuse injuries and boredom. It involves using a workout schedule that alternates days for a variety of fitness activities.

Diastolic pressure is the blood pressure within the arteries when the heart is in relaxation between contractions.

Duration is the length of time devoted to an exercise or an exercise session.

Eccentric contraction is when a muscle elongates as it contracts, as when a weight is gradually lowered and the contracting muscle(s) elongate(s) as it/they release(s) the tension.

Ectomorph is a somatotype (body type) describing a person who appears thin and lean.

Eddy resistance is the drag that occurs as the body moves through water. Clothing worn over bathing suits, resistance equipment, and bent limbs moving through the water will bring about increased eddy resistance.

Empty calories refer to calories yielded by food that are void or nearly void of nutrients, protein, vitamins, and minerals. This usually refers to foods having high sugar or fat content, and alcoholic beverages.

Endomorph is a somatotype (body type) describing a person who appears soft and round with a predominance of fat tissue, but who is not necessarily obese.

Evaporation is heat lost through the evaporation of moisture from the skin (perspiration, splashed-on water) as air flows over it.

Extension is increasing the angle of a joint (e.g., straightening your arms from a bent position).

Fat, a compound containing glycerol and fatty acids, is stored in the body as adipose tissue. It serves as a concentrated source of energy for muscular work.

Fatigue refers to a diminished capacity for work as a result of prolonged or excessive exertion.

Flexibility is the ability of a joint to move through its full range of motion.

Flexion is the bending of a joint between two bones that decreases the angle between the two bones.

High-impact is a form of exercise that incorporates jumping and bouncing movements. There is a high degree of impact placed on the joints, bones, and feet in this form of aerobic exercise.

Hyperextension occurs when the angle of a joint is moved past the normal range of motion.

Hypothermia is defined as a depression in core temperature sufficient to affect bodily functions, usually below 95° Fahrenheit.

Inertia refers to the resistance of the body to any change of motion. An object will remain either stationary or moving unless acted upon by an outside force.

Inertia lag is the loss of forward momentum, which will require extra energy to be expended to put the body back into motion.

Intensity is the level of difficulty of an exercise or workout.

Interval training combines segments of high-intensity aerobic training with periods of low-intensity aerobic training.

Isometric muscle contraction is a contraction of the muscle without the movement of a limb. An example of this is when you push the palms of your hands together in front of your chest to contract your biceps and pectoralis muscles.

Isotonic muscle contraction is when the muscle changes length to move a body part or an object, as in weight training.

Low impact is a form of exercise that does not jar the body very much. In the land-type dance-exercise class this refers to keeping one foot on the floor at all times; it often refers to aerobic classes that involve no jumping or that are done in the shallow end of a swimming pool.

Low intensity means a reduced workload, or working at a lower target heart rate.

Mesomorph is a somatotype (body type) describing a very muscular, athletic-looking individual.

Metabolism is the chemical reaction of a cell or living tissue that transfers usable materials into energy.

Muscular endurance is the ability of the muscles to exert force over an extended period of time.

Muscular strength is the amount of force produced when a muscle group contracts and moves a resistance.

Muzak is a term popularly used to refer to background music that one may have playing but to which one is not listening carefully. It may be considered musical background noise.

Nautilus is a type of weight machine that uses special cams to change the amount of force needed to lift the weight so that the muscle is working closer to its maximum ability throughout the exercise.

Overload is the method used to increase one's workload beyond the normal capacity in order to improve and develop muscular strength and endurance.

Overuse syndrome refers to nagging, slow-to-heal ailments that result from exercising too much too soon; it can involve muscles, tendons, or bones and responds to a treatment of rest, ice, compression, and elevation (RICE).

Perceived exertion is a means of measuring how hard one is exercising by comparing a subjective self-rating with an established chart of various levels.

Plumbline is a weighted string that is held at a specific point on the body to demark a straight line through a plane of the body. To check correct posture, it is held at the mastoid process to mark a line through the sagittal plane of the body.

Pronation is the rotation of the bone/body part toward the midline of the body.

Prone is lying face down.

Radial artery is the artery located on the inside of the wrist. It lies very close to the surface of the skin and, therefore, is often used for counting one's pulse.

Radiation is the absorption of heat energy to and from solid objects. An example is body temperature increasing from the sun.

Recovery heart rate is how quickly your pulse returns to normal after an aerobic workout.

Repetition is one complete action of an exercise.

Resting heart rate refers to the number of times your heart beats per minute when you have been sitting or resting for approximately 10 minutes.

RICE is the acronym for rest, ice, compression, elevation (the steps for immediate injury treatment).

Risk factors are genetic and nongenetic characteristics that contribute to the incidence of heart disease or stroke.

Scull or sculling is small motions initiated by the arms and hands. It is sometimes thought of as a Figure 8-type motion. When performed laterally, the cue is thumbs up, thumbs down. When performed moving toward the thighs, it could be palms in, palms out.

Set(s) refers to a sequence of movements. For example, you may repeat a particular movement three times, which would comprise one set.

Set-point theory proposes that the human metabolism works very hard to maintain a certain body weight; that weight is held in place through complex homeostatic mechanisms.

Shin splints is a catch-all phrase used to describe any discomfort in the front lower leg. It is usually a result of overuse syndrome.

Side stitch refers to a pain in the side during exercise. It is thought to be caused by a spasm in the diaphragm, due to insufficient oxygen supply and improper breathing.

Sprain refers to a wrenching or twisting of a joint in which ligaments are stretched past their normal limits.

Static stretching movements place the muscle in a sustained stretch position for a given period of time. This is an effective way to achieve flexibility in a specific muscle group. It is the opposite of ballistic stretching movements.

Stationary inertia is what an aquatic exerciser must overcome when initiating movement from a motionless position in shallow water.

Strain refers to a muscle pull—a stretch or tear of the muscle or adjacent tissue.

Strength is the maximum force or tension that a muscle or muscle group can produce against a resistance.

Supination is the rotation of a bone/body part away from the midline of the body.

Supine is lying face up.

Target heart rate is the level at which you will gain the benefits of exercising your heart to improve cardiovascular fitness.

Tempo is the rate of speed of a musical piece or passage.

Tendinitis is inflammation of a tendon; it often requires several weeks of rest to heal completely.

Tendon is a band of dense, fibrous tissue forming the termination of a muscle and attaching muscle to bone with a minimum of elasticity.

Thermoregulation is the body's attempt to maintain a constant core temperature.

Time refers to the length of time devoted to a workout, a class, or a particular exercise.

Training effects are the physiologic adaptations that occur as a result of aerobic exercise of sufficient intensity, frequency, and duration to produce beneficial changes in the body.

Triglycerides are compounds composed of glycerol fatty acids. They are stored in the body and are unhealthy when present in high levels.

Vein is a vessel that carries blood away from the body and toward the heart.

Ventricle is a lower lobe of the heart. There is a right ventricle and a left ventricle.

Vertebrae are the bony or cartilaginous segments that are separated by discs and make up the spinal column.

Warm-up is a balanced combination of static-stretch and rhythmic-limbering exercises that prepares the body for more vigorous exercise.

Working heart rate is the heart rate taken at the end of the aerobic section of a workout to identify whether the individual was working in his/her target heart rate zone and at the proper intensity for his/her age and physical fitness level.

Zero (no) impact exercise refers to exercise performed in the deep end of a swimming pool, or while buoyantly supported in the water, which places no strain or weight on the bones, joints, tendons, or muscles.

INDEX